MATERNITY IN IRELAND

A Woman-Centred Perspective

Patricia Kennedy

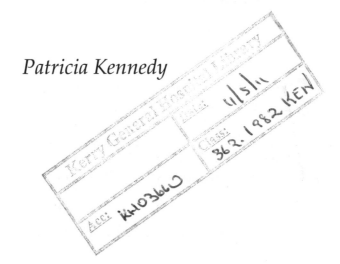

The Liffey Press
Dublin

Published by
The Liffey Press Ltd
Ashbrook House, 10 Main Street
Raheny, Dublin 5, Ireland
www.theliffeypress.com

A catalogue record of this book is
available from the British Library.

ISBN 1-904148-16-6

The author and publishers are grateful for support from the Academic
Publications Scheme administered by the Office of Funded Research
Support Services at University College Dublin.

Printed in the Republic of Ireland by Colour Books Ltd.

ABOUT THE AUTHOR

Patricia Kennedy PhD is a Senior Lecturer in the Department of Social Policy and Social Work in University College Dublin. She is a founder member of the Irish Social Policy Association. She is co-editor of *Irish Social Policy in Context* and *Contemporary Irish Social Policy* (University College Dublin Press, 1999). She is co-author of *Returning Birth to Women: Challenging Policies and Practice* and is sole author of *Domestic Violence: The Tallaght Experience*. She recently co-authored, on behalf of the Women's Health Unit of the Northern Area Health Board, a major research report on the *Maternity Needs of Refugees and Asylum Seeking Women*; and co-authored a research report: *A Survey of Users' Views and Perceptions of Symptomatic Breast Care Services* for the Women's Health Council. She has also published articles on Traveller women; the criminal justice system; and the social economy. She represented the National Women's Council of Ireland on the Kinder Review of Maternity Services in the North Eastern Health Board and is currently a member of the North Eastern Health Board Task Force on Maternity Services.

CONTENTS

ACKNOWLEDGEMENTS

I would like to thank all of the people who made the completion of this book possible. Over the years I have met hundreds of women who have shared their birth experiences with me, which has informed my thinking on maternity. I am grateful to all of the health professionals who shared their experiences and very valuable time with me, especially those in the National Maternity Hospital, the Coombe Women's Hospital, the Rotunda Hospital and in the North Eastern Health Board. I would like to thank all of the NGOs that supplied me with very valuable information, particularly the Home Birth Association, Cuidiú and the La Leche League. I would like to give special thanks to the many people who have helped me with statistical data over the years, particularly those in the Central Statistics Office, the Department of Social, Community and Family Affairs, the Eastern Region Health Authority and the Department of Health and Children. Thanks also to the library staff in UCD, both in Belfield and Earlsfort Terrace, and to Michael Foley in the National Disability Authority, Noreen Geoghegan in Cherry Orchard Hospital, Geraldine Lambe (PHN) in Benburb Street and all those associated with the Women's Health Unit at the Northern Area Health Authority. I am grateful to Professor John Bonnar for sharing his wealth of experience and expertise with me.

Special thanks goes to Professor Gabriel Kiely and all of the staff of the Department of Social Policy and Social Work at UCD, for their constant patience, encouragement and support. I am particularly grateful to Professor Helen Burke and Dr Pauline Conroy for their guidance over the years while I completed my doctoral thesis on which this book is largely based. I am indebted to Jo Murphy-Lawless and Anne Coakley for all of their expert advice but more importantly their friendship. I would like to thank Mary Alyward, Olivia Carr, Liz Hickey, and Helen Smith for their constant support and friendship; Sharon and Karen for loving and minding my children so that I was free to write this book; Gary Collins for his guidance and wisdom; and Kate Spillane for teaching me how empowering the experience of childbirth can be. Thanks to Brian Langan and David Givens of The Liffey Press for all of their hard work in the publication of this book.

Finally I would like to dedicate this book to Mick, Conor, Dylan, Fionn and Millie, who have taught me both the joys and challenges of motherhood.

GLOSSARY

Adrenalin: a hormone secreted by the adrenalin gland, which prepares the body for "fight or flight", has effects on circulation and muscles.

Age-specific fertility rate: the number of live births to women in that age group per 1,000 females in the same age group.

Amniocentesis: withdrawal of a sample of the amniotic fluid surrounding an embryo in the uterus by piercing the amniotic sac through the abdominal wall. This enables chromosomal patterns to be studied so that chromosomal abnormalities can be detected.

Amniotic sac: an oval bag inside the uterus consisting of two thin membranes.

Caesarean section: a surgical operation for delivering a baby through the abdominal wall. The lower uterine caesarean section (LUCS) is carried out through an incision in the lower segment of the uterus. In a classical caesarean section (CSS), the upper segment of the uterus is incised.

Cervix: the neck of the uterus, which gradually opens up during labour.

Chorionic Villus sampling (CVS): a fetal monitoring technique in which a sample of chorionic villus is taken between the eight and eleventh weeks of pregnancy. Sampling is carried out through the cervix or abdomen under ultrasound visualisation. This enables the prenatal diagnosis of congenital disorders, through chromosomal and biochemical studies.

Colostrum: the secretion from the nipples that precedes lactation.

Contractions: regular tightening of the muscles of the uterus. During labour, these become more forceful and will push the baby down the birth canal.

Embryo: the baby is referred to as an embryo in the early stages of pregnancy, usually the first six weeks.

Engaged: the baby's head drops down into the pelvis so that the widest part of its head is through the pelvic brim. This usually occurs at around 36 weeks in a first pregnancy and later in subsequent pregnancies.

Epidural analgesia: a local anaesthetic injected into the epidural space around the spinal sac, causing loss of sensations to the lower part of the body.

Episiotomy: surgical cut to the perineum to expedite delivery.

Expected date of delivery (EDD): the expected date of birth.

Extremely very low birth weight (EVLBW): less than 1,000 grams.

Fetus: the baby is referred to as a fetus from seven weeks.

Gestation: the period from conception to birth.

Iatrogenic: a condition that has resulted from treatment, as either an unforeseen or inevitable side effect.

Induction: any process which starts labour artificially.

Infant mortality: liveborns surviving less than one year.

Intra Uterine Growth Retardation (IUGR): the condition resulting in the birth of a baby with a weight on or below the weight predicted gestational age.

Lithotomy: birth position lying on one's back.

Live birth: defined in the perinatal statistics as: ". . . the complete expulsion or extraction from its mother of a product of conception, irrespective of the duration of pregnancy, which after such separation, breathes or shows any other evidence of life, such as beating of the heart, pulsation of the umbilical cord, or definite movement of voluntary muscles, whether or not the umbilical cord has been cut or the placenta is attached" (Department of Health, 1991: 12). In accordance with the WHO guidelines, live births weighing less than 500 grams are not included in the national statistics.

Lochia: the material eliminated from the uterus via the vagina after childbirth.

Low birth weight: less than 2,500 grams.

Maternal mortality: defined as the death of a woman while pregnant or within 42 days of termination of pregnancy.

Meconium: the first stools of a newborn baby which are sticky and dark green and composed of cellular debris, mucus and bile pigments. The presence of meconium in the amniotic fluid during labour can be an indication of fetal distress.

Miscarriage: broadly defined as the expulsion of the embryo or fetus before viability has been achieved.

Morbidity: the state of being diseased.

Multigravida: a woman who has been pregnant at least twice.

Neonatal mortality: liveborns surviving less than four weeks.

Noradrenalin: a substance of adrenalin.

Oxytocin: a hormone released by the pituitary gland, which causes contraction of the uterus during labour and stimulates milk flow from the breasts by causing contraction of muscles.

Perinatal mortality: liveborns surviving less than one week plus late fetals (after 28 weeks of pregnancy). Figures refer to the definition of late fetal deaths at or over 28 weeks gestation. From 1995 in CSO statistics, there is a new broader definition of stillbirths at over 500 grams or at a gestational age of 24 weeks or more. (Table 4.19 uses the older definition for purposes of comparison.)

Perineum: the area of pelvic floor between vagina and pelvis.

Pethidine: an analgesic drug with mild sedative action, used to relieve moderate or severe pain. It is administered by mouth or injection; side-effects may include nausea and dizziness .

Placenta: an organ within the uterus by means of which the embryo is attached to the wall of the uterus. It provides nourishment, eliminates wastes and exchanges respiratory gases.

Primagravida: a woman pregnant for the first time.

Primapara: a woman pregnant for the first time.

Prontosil: an antibiotic.

Puerperal infection: infection of the female genital tract arising as a complication of childbirth.

Puerperal pyrexia: a temperature of 38°C occurring on any two days within 14 days of childbirth or miscarriage.

Puerperium: the period of up to about six weeks after childbirth, during which the uterus returns to its original size.

Syntocinon: a pituitary extract used to induce uterine contractions and to control or prevent postpartum haemorrhage.

TENS: transcutaneous electrical nerve stimulation, the introduction of pulses of low voltage electricity into tissue for relief of pain.

Total period fertility rate (TPFR): a theoretical concept, it is the average number of children that would be born alive to a woman during her lifetime if she were to pass through her childbearing years (15–49) conforming to the age-specific fertility rates of a given year. The TPFR is calculated by adding the age-specific fertility rates for the relevant five-year age groups, dividing by 1,000 and multiplying by five.

Toxaemia: blood poisoning that is caused by bacteria growing in a local site of infection. It produces generalised symptoms including fever, diarrhoea and vomiting.

Trimester: pregnancy is divided into three trimesters; the first is the first thirteen weeks of pregnancy, the second lasts from 14 to 27 weeks and the third is from week 28 until delivery.

Ultrasound scan (USS): a highly sophisticated instrument which uses soundwaves to show the development of the baby in the uterus.

Umbilical cord: the link between the baby and the mother (placenta). Blood circulates through the cord carrying oxygen and food to the baby and removing waste.

Very low birth weight (VLBW): less than 1,500 grams.

Chapter One

INTRODUCTION

All human life on the planet is born of woman. The one unifying, uncontrollable experience shared by all women and men is that months-long period we spent unfolding inside a woman's body. Because young humans remain dependent upon nurture for a much longer period than other mammals, and because of the division of labour long established in human groups, where women not only bear and suckle but are assigned almost total responsibility for children, most of us know both love and disappointment, power and tenderness in the person of a woman. We carry the imprint of this experience for life, even into dying. Yet there has been a strange lack of material to help us understand and use it (Rich, 1977: 11).

Despite the fact that in excess of 50,000 women in Ireland give birth each year, and many more experience pregnancy, there has been a huge lacuna in the analysis of social policies which directly affect women during this period of their lives. This book is an attempt to rectify this omission. It focuses on Irish health, welfare and labour market policies which directly affect women during pregnancy and the first year of motherhood, that is: "the maternity period". These policies reflect the three dimensions of a woman's life when pregnant and childbearing, when a woman must combine lifegiving, caring and earning. These three roles are lived out in the context of health, welfare and labour market policies. Motherhood is both personal and political. Mothers live their lives where the public and private meet. Their everyday lives are influenced by public expectations, prescribed roles, social, political, economic, and cultural constraints and circumstances while on a parallel level private, biographical, emotional, physical and psychological experiences have to be coped with by these same mothers. While acknowledging that mothers' and infants' welfare are inextricably linked, the focus of this book is on mothers.

MOTHERHOOD AS AN INSTITUTION AND AS BIOLOGICAL PROCESS

> I did not understand that this circle, this magnetic field in which we lived, was not a natural phenomenon (Rich, 1980: 4–5).

Rich in *Of Woman Born* traces the development of motherhood as an institution distinguishing between biological motherhood and motherhood as an institution. The latter she claims is subject to male control and "has been a keystone of the most diverse social and political systems" (1977: 13). Jackson (1994) suggests that mothering as we know it is actually a specific institution, which has been constructed and defined historically and its very form changes according to changing economic and political needs. Atkinson, referring to "motherhood, the ancient vocation that is also an institution" (1991: *ix*), examines the social construction of motherhood asking how have "good" and "bad" motherhood been constructed. She argues that motherhood is socially constructed both historically and culturally, based on assumptions regarding the physiology of motherhood and that "what is known and believed about conception, pregnancy, birth and lactation not only describes what mothers are but colors expectations of what they should be" (1991: 21). She outlines how medicine has traditionally defined women as mothers whether or not they have children, "as walking (or wandering) wombs". She examines how from Plato onwards women were classified by both male scientists and philosophers as different, as the other, as non-male "with different reproductive organs and systems. Aristotle defined gender in terms of reproductive potential and identified femaleness itself with reproductive deficiency" (1991: 238). This view was transferred into the nineteenth and twentieth centuries via Thomas Aquinas. Atkinson indicates that twentieth-century developments in reproductive technology challenge social theory and ethics: "who is a mother; the donor of an ovum, the woman who carries a fetus to term, or the person who raises a son or daughter to maturity" (1991: 24). Van Buren suggests that:

> Each culture or society organises mothering, pregnancy, birth and child care to fit the economics, religion and scientific beliefs of that time and place. Moreover, whatever the pattern or structure, the emotional origins of the madonna and child configuration lie within themes of survival, potency and mortality (1989: 1).

Oakley identifies how motherhood in relation to feminism has had different issues stressed at different times. Such issues have ranged from access to home births to access to abortion: "what has tended to happen is that feminists have used a particular and (class-differentiated) vision of the status quo in order to define a different projected future for motherhood" (1986a: 128). Motherhood and feminism have to be examined historically. Oakley traces the relationship between feminism and motherhood from the eighteenth and early nineteenth centuries, arguing that during those centuries the focus was on the political, economic and psychological effects of women's enforced dependency on men rather than on the health aspects of motherhood.

In the nineteenth and early twentieth centuries, according to Oakley, feminism stated a variety of positions about motherhood:

> . . . the struggle to render women citizens overshadowed the need to understand motherhood in relation to women's overall situation, psychology or future as differentiated by class, ethnicity and economics. Motherhood remained essentially unproblematic (1986a: 131).

Problems perceived to be associated with women's situation were, according to Oakley, associated with the law, government, education and citizenship. She credits the increasing influence of medicine over motherhood as a reason for feminists moving their attention to motherhood:

> . . . medicine, under the title of the maternal and child health movement, was beginning to colonize a new area of women's lives, at a time at which the theoretical and practical significance of this area to women's position as a whole had scarcely been grasped by anyone (1986a: 132).

She links this interest in maternal and infant health to capitalism and the concern with public health and a belief that public health was something which could be managed. Oakley claims that "the period from the 1920s to the 1960s is a particularly interesting one from the point of view of the dialectic between feminism and medicine on the topic of motherhood" (1986a: 135).

BIOLOGICAL ESSENTIALISM

Sayers introduces a very important argument to the social construction debate about motherhood. She distinguishes between social constructionism and biological essentialism, arguing that what is needed within feminist debate is "a third position . . . which takes issue with both biological essentialism and social constructionism" (1982: 3). She argues that social constructionism is an inadequate alternative to biological essentialism and argues that "sexual inequality has been determined by biological as well as social and historical factors". Furthermore, she suggests that this was the "position adopted in early psychoanalytic and Marxist accounts of sexual divisions in society" (1982: 4). Sayers examines how the various strands of contemporary feminism incorporate biology into their analyses. Acknowledging that to adequately classify contemporary feminism is problematic, Sayers offers four ideological approaches: liberalism, Marxism, radical and socialist feminism. Sayers refers to the work of liberal writers like Archer (1976) who suggests that social inequalities are not linked to biological differences but rather to sexual discrimination. Regarding Marxist feminists, Sayers draws on the work of classical Marxists to argue that essentially they "assert that social factors are prior to biological factors in determining women's social status" (1982: 187). Sayers argues that socialist feminism has emerged out of a discontent with Marxist feminism, referring in particular to the fact that sexual divisions have continued to exist within the family even in socialist countries. Regarding radical feminism, Sayers, referring to the work of Firestone (1979), Rich (1977) and Daly (1978), claims that they view biology as central to sexual divisions and discrimination in society. Sayers concludes that "the answers to the woman question are not to be found solely in biology" (1982: 187) and I, together with many other feminist writers, would agree with her.

MOTHERHOOD AND SOCIAL POLICY

This book focuses on the point where mothers' roles as carer, earner and lifegiver intersect. I argue that this is the very point where mothers' lives are articulated. It is the nexus where the private and public domains of a mother's life meet and thus is of crucial significance to feminist theory, to social policy, to society and to families. As women are commonly perceived in society as "potential mothers", and their place and status within society is very much shaped by this perception, this will contribute to an understanding of the organisation of welfare as it affects all women. Leira, in her study of mothers in Scandinavia, argues that while not all women personally experience motherhood, almost all women in society are affected by its potentiality (1992: 3). Data for Ireland show that 79 per cent of women do in fact become mothers (O'Connor, 1995).

In recent years there has emerged in Ireland the beginnings of a rich body of literature on women's experiences within society. This has come from a variety of sources, influenced undoubtedly by the women's movement and the development of women's studies within the major universities, the increased involvement of women in employment and in community-based initiatives and the increasingly visible linkages between women's organisations across Europe, as Ireland has become part of a greater European Union. Such studies have been shaped by a variety of academic disciplines and theories and provide a valuable insight into the context in which women live their lives. Internationally, feminist social policy has so far concerned itself with mothers as workers and as carers and many writers in recent years have devoted much time and attention to policies affecting particular groups of mothers, for example, lone mothers. There has been a very serious lack of attention in Ireland to policies which relate specifically to the health of women as they experience pregnancy, childbirth and the postpartum period. This is a serious omission in the light of the failings in health services that have emerged in recent years, which directly and seriously affected the lives of pregnant women. These include the Hepatitis C scandal and the allegations against a consultant obstetrician in relation to excessive use of caesarean hysterectomy at Our Lady of Lourdes Hospital in Drogheda. Childbirth in Ireland has become more medicalised as smaller maternity units have closed since the 1970s. This has happened without much discussion or debate by anyone other than local community activists. Social policy analysts have not been involved in any discourse on this subject.

In an Irish context, any analysis of health policies relating to the maternity period have come from sociologists, to the forefront of whom is Murphy-Lawless (1987, 1992a, 1992b, 1998a, 1998b) joined in recent years by MacAdam-O'Connell (1998) and O'Connor (1992, 1995, 1998) and childbirth educators such as Mason (1995, 1998). Any other analysis has come from childbirth activists, for example, O'Regan (1998), Martin (1998) and Dunlop (1998). An even subtler gap in the social policy literature is the dearth of analysis regarding the association between women's physiological experience of pregnancy and childbirth and how these are intertwined with mothers' everyday lives as carers and as earners. This book, therefore, endeavours to break new ground in terms of policy analysis by examining policies in Ireland, which relate to the lived experiences of women as they labour in childbirth, in caring and in the labour market. Oakley (1986a: 127) states that at each point in history there tends to be a dominant definition of motherhood, which stresses a "right" way to be a mother. It is hoped that this book will illuminate the dominant model of motherhood which has developed in the Irish context and been reinforced by social policies.

Mothers, for the most part, have been rendered invisible, or when visible have been seen one-dimensionally, either as carers or earners, dividing the private realm of unpaid work from the public realm of paid work. Leira has taken a two-dimensional approach looking at mothers' roles as carer/earner. This approach according to Leira "shows that the remaking of motherhood is generated by welfare state policies and by mothers' everyday practices" (1992: 5). Leira argues that the analysis of motherhood has to take place within a broad context:

> . . . which makes explicit the different ways in which the welfare state has dealt with economic provision and caring respectively, as activities of individuals, how caring and earning are integrated into the welfare state benefit and entitlement system? Which social rights do earning and caring give access to? What do caring and earning entail in a citizenship perspective? Is there such a thing as citizen the carer? (1992: 5).

Motherhood as Multi-dimensional

While Leira has developed a very useful model for understanding mothers' relationship to the welfare state, I would argue that Leira's contribution, while significant, is still inadequate. Since women primarily find themselves in the role of carers, and many juggle this with their role as earners, this study would argue that both of these roles could be passed on to other parties, be it the State, other women, friends or relations. However, there is another dimension to women's role as mother which cannot be passed on. This is the physiological dimension. It is only woman who can conceive, lactate and give birth. It is only the birth mother who is caught in the grips of labour pain. It is she who lies under the abortionist, suffers the pain of a miscarriage or the ecstasy or trauma of birth. It is only the physiological mother who lactates. These are the basic elements which a woman has to balance with her role as carer and earner, and these are the most crucial issues so often ignored by social policy analysts. This is the area of a woman's life deemed as private and as such outside the sphere of social policy. However, such essentially private areas as contraception and abortion have been commandeered by the media, legislators and the Church as public issues. O'Brien reminds us that "it is from an adequate understanding of the process of reproduction, nature's traditional and bitter trap for the suppression of women, that women can begin to understand their possibilities and their freedom" (1981: 8). In this book, I develop a three-dimensional model of motherhood in an attempt to understand this process in the Irish context (Figure 1.1).

Figure 1.1: A Three Dimensional Model of Motherhood — Mother as Carer, Earner and Lifegiver

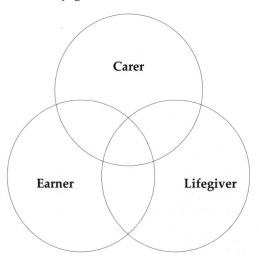

METHODOLOGY

I draw on feminist writings, theories and perspectives:

> Feminism means finally that we renounce our obedience of
> the fathers and recognise the world they have described is not
> the whole world. Masculine ideologies are the creation of
> masculine subjectivity, they are neither objective or value-free,
> nor inclusively "human". Feminism implies that we recognise
> fully the inadequacy for us, the distortion, of male centered
> ideologies and that we proceed to think and act out of that
> recognition (Rich, 1980: 20).

Reinharz refers to the use of "multiple methods" in feminist schol-
arship (1992: 197). This book makes use of documentary analysis,
statistical data and women's birth accounts, arguing that "multi-
method research creates the opportunity to put texts or people in
contexts, thus providing a richer and far more accurate
interpretation" (Reinharz, 1992: 213). There is much scholarly debate regarding the methods of feminist research. While feminist
writers often employ qualitative methods and stress the importance of biography, I agree with Reinharz that "feminism is a perspective, not a method" (Reinharz, 1992: 241) and that:

> . . . feminism supplies the perspective and the disciplines sup-
> ply the method . . . feminist researchers adopt the methods of
> their discipline without any major modification. They use a
> discipline for its power turning its power to feminist ends
> (Reinharz, 1992: 243).

Thus, I adopt the use of documentary and statistical analysis
while incorporating a feminist perspective. But to what "feminist
ends" are these methods directed to achieve? I agree with Roberts
(1981) who claims that the duty of feminist research is threefold.
First, it must criticise existing social structures and ways of per-
ceiving them. Secondly, it must introduce corrective mechanisms
by providing an alternative viewpoint and data to substantiate it.
Thirdly, it must start to lay groundwork for a transformation of

social science and society. These are the aims of this researcher with regard to pregnancy and maternity policies in Ireland.

This book draws on official documents relevant to health policy, in particular maternity policies, labour and social welfare legislation and policy documents, both Irish and European. It analyses discussion documents, which are often an important resource. An analysis of the clinical reports of the three principal maternity hospitals in Dublin — the Coombe Women's Hospital (formerly the Coombe-Lying-In Hospital), the Rotunda and the National Maternity Hospital (Holles Street) — are a valuable resource for demonstrating the changing birthing patterns and intervention rates in Irish maternity units. Statistical trends from the annual clinical reports of the three hospitals, where over 40 per cent of all Irish births occur, for the 30-year period from 1970–2000 are examined. The research also draws on statistical reports from the Department of Social, Community and Family Affairs, the Department of Health and Children, the Central Statistics Office and Eurostat.

I draw largely on the work of Enkin et al. (2000), *A Guide to Effective Care in Pregnancy and Childbirth* (third edition). In 1980, the authors began to assemble a register of controlled trials in perinatal medicine and what developed was the systematic review of the effects of care during pregnancy and childbirth, which forms the basis of their book. Criteria were identified which would provide the best evidence to evaluate care, utilising the Mediline database as well as hand searches from over 60 key journals since 1950. Over 40,000 obstetricians in 18 countries were written to in an attempt to identify unpublished studies. What emerged was a systematic synthesis of all of these methods. The result was *Effective Care in Pregnancy and Childbirth*, a 1,500-page book in two large volumes and a database of reviews. The latter is now incorporated in the Cochrane database of systematic reviews and is available on disc as *The Cochrane Pregnancy and Childbirth Database.* Enkin et al. (2000) is an attempt to make the findings of the larger publications more accessible to all involved in the care of childbearing women. The 1997 Report of the Audit Commission (UK)

refers to the Cochrane database as having "broadened the definitions applied to outcomes of care and offered clinicians a wider
grasp of maternity-related research" (1997: 5).

OUTLINE OF THIS BOOK

The book begins by explaining the medical and social models of
childbirth. It then goes on to look at some of the most salient factors in relation to the development of maternity policies for
women in Ireland between Independence and 1970. This is followed by a more detailed exploration of policy developments between 1970 and 2000. It presents statistical data to challenge
myths which have developed in Ireland in relation to fertility
trends. It draws on statistics to demonstrate the extent to which a
medical model rather than a social model of childbirth has become dominant in Ireland. As there are now more potential users
of maternity services than at any time since 1970, it explores implications for consumers, policy-makers and service providers.
The increased hospitalisation, and thus management, of childbirth
has led to an increased dependency on expensive labour-intensive
technology. As the numbers of births rise there is potentially a
greater demand for direct maternity and infant care as well as
wider social support services. During the 1970 to 2000 period, the
number of women giving birth for the first time aged under 25
and over 35 years have both decreased, changing the age profile
of mothers and shortening the period in which women are likely
to give birth to the ten-year period between 25 and 35 years. This
also has implications for planners, as research presented in this
book demonstrates that women in this age group are less likely to
give birth to babies of low birth weight, which places an extra
demand on services. One of the most significant changes in terms
of outcome of birth is the decline in maternal mortality from 17
per 100,000 in 1971 to two per 100,000 in 2000 with a corresponding decline in perinatal, neonatal and infant mortality. These patterns are important as they are often interpreted as evidence that
the increased hospitalisation of childbirth, as well as higher rates

of intervention, have been responsible for this improvement in outcome. This debate is further explored later in this book. This analysis of statistical patterns relating to pregnancy and maternity has raised some important issues not only in relation to health policies but also in relation to welfare and labour market policies, and these too are examined in the following chapters.

Women are not a homogenous group. Therefore, as women progress through the maternity period some may have additional or specific needs. For example, there are needs which are specific to disabled women, women from the Traveller community and women from other ethnic groups who may have come to Ireland seeking asylum. Another group of women with very specific medical and social support needs are women who are using or may have previously used illegal drugs. This book addresses these important issues.

As more mothers are now active in the labour market, rights to maternity, paternity and parental leave have become contested issues. These are discussed in Chapters Eleven and Twelve, when women's three-dimensional roles as carer, earner and lifegiver are brought together in the context of developing comprehensive woman-centred maternity provision for all women.

Chapter Two

THE MEDICAL AND SOCIAL MODELS OF CHILDBIRTH

Central to this book is a belief that women must have power and control over their own sexuality and reproductive capacities and that they must be guaranteed dignity and respect throughout every stage of pregnancy, delivery and the postpartum period. This chapter is concerned with the physiological aspect of women's lives and it argues that childbirth must be "woman-centered". A British report, *Changing Childbirth*, recognises the principles of good woman-centred care as:

> The woman must be the focus of maternity care. She should be able to feel that she is in control of what is happening to her and able to make decisions about her care, based on her needs, having discussed maternity fully with the professionals involved.

> Maternity services must be readily and easily accessible to all. They should be sensitive to the needs of the local population and based primarily in the community.

> Women should be involved in the monitoring and planning of maternity services to ensure that they are responsive to the needs of a changing society. In addition care should be effective and resources used efficiently (Department of Health, Great Britain, 1993: 8).

This book extends these principles to an overarching concept that includes welfare and labour market policies, arguing that all policies which affect a woman during pregnancy and the first year of motherhood must be woman-centred.

Currently, there are two schools of thought underlying Irish maternal health care provision. The principal model dominant in maternity units is what is known as the "active management of labour", and is best presented in the textbook for obstetric students in Ireland of the same name (O'Driscoll et al., 1993). The book, first published in 1982, is in its third edition and the authors between them have served as Masters to the National Maternity Hospital for almost 20 years. A fourth edition is due out in the summer of 2003 but is not associated with the current personnel of the National Maternity Hospital. The third edition, published in 1993, however serves as a historical document to show how this philosophy has become so dominant. The authors of the 1993 edition tell us that they:

> . . . were directly responsible for 100,000 births and who for the intervening years were closely involved with an additional 100,000 births — a total of some 200,000 births overall. The text encompasses a comprehensive approach to the conduct of labour as put into effect several times every day in one of the largest obstetric units in the British Isles (p. 13).

Active management of labour is currently a near blanket practice in Irish maternity, as data presented in this book demonstrates. Murphy-Lawless refers to the active management of labour as:

> . . . a mode of organisation whereby the consultant obstetrician became actively involved in the conduct of labour on an ongoing basis as never before with the delivery unit of the hospital redesignated as an intensive-care unit (1998a: 25).

Murphy-Lawless continues: ". . . when we are reading the clinical records, textbooks and debates, the assertions and contentions of Irish obstetrics, we are reading our own history as Irish women of institutionalised childbirth" (1998a: 25). She describes:

> A system of hospitalised birth, which has been fostered by the National Maternity Hospital and exported world-wide, hun-

dreds and thousands of textbooks and thousands of articles have marked out a distinctive Irish contribution to obstetrics, a contribution which has implicated thousands of Irish women (1998a: 25).

At the other end of the spectrum there exists what is referred to as "active birth" and is best presented in the writings of Balaskas (1979), Kitzinger (1978, 1988, 1993), Odent (1984) and Leboyer (1975, 1991) and is identified in Ireland with those claiming the right to have a "natural birth" either in a maternity unit or at home. Wagner argues that behind the social and medical approaches to childbirth there lies "a set of assumptions, ideas and thinking" (1994: 27). He stresses that he is not concerned with labeling one model right and another wrong, but rather "to explore how to combine them by identifying the elements in each that might be effective in addressing specific health issues". Wagner (1994: 27) explains how the conflict between the two models dates from ancient Greek philosophy but has become deeply ingrained in Western thought. They relate to the dichotomised world which views art and all that is subjective, feminine, based on intuition and quality on one side, while on the other there exists science, objectivity, masculinity, logic and quantity. He claims that before the modern era, health and birth were related to the artistic side, the social model, whereas:

> About a hundred years ago, the profession of medicine aligned itself with science and classical, mechanical physics, applying them to the body, its functions and its disease processes: this was the basis for the medical model of health. As pregnancy and birth were brought into the medical domain this view was applied to birth and birth technology (1994: 27–28).

Murphy-Lawless argues that:

> Obstetrics is a medical specialism and, even though it has an exclusive focus on the female body, it has strategies of knowledge production and organisation similar to other branches of medical science. Similar to the rest of Western biomedicine,

obstetrics presents specific social realities as a "natural given", bundling them into what is then presented as a scientifically proven basis for its practices (1998a: 32–33).

The period from conception to childbirth is a period which reflects the public/private divisions of women's lives. Conception is a result of an intimate private act. However, the nine months following conception are a long journey for a woman as she travels in and out of the public world of hospital appointments and the public gaze and comments as her body blooms and grows, and the private, silent world of morning sickness, exhaustion and feelings of loneliness, isolation and at other times happiness, even ecstasy. For some there is the private loss of miscarriage and for an increasing number of Irish women pregnancy ends in termination. For others the journey ends with a stillborn baby. The journey into the patriarchal world of medicine and eventually birth for the majority of women takes place in a very public, male-controlled labour ward (Oakley, 1979, 1980, 1992; Tew, 1995). On the way to this ward women undergo a period of socialisation and education as they attend ante-natal appointments and classes (Mason, 1995, 1998).

> Birth is an isolated biological episode only to hospital administrators and official statisticians; the women who give birth have a past and a future. So it is in this biographical context that childbirth has its social meaning (Oakley, 1979: 23).

Pregnancy, and in particular a first-time pregnancy (Oakley, 1979), can be a lonely, alienating and frightening experience for many women. In modern society, it has tended to take on major significance as a "rite of passage" for women. It is a life-changing experience, through which one's status, role and responsibility within society change. Oakley indicates that first-time motherhood in particular requires a woman to make enormous changes in her life so that:

> . . . becoming a mother is more than a change of job, it involves reorganising one's entire personality. For there is a chasm be-

tween mothers' needs and children's needs that mothers have
to bridge (1979: 12).

LEARNING TO DISTINGUISH BETWEEN THE SOCIAL AND MEDICAL MODELS

> For the newborn child to enter our world is to enter a realm of
> opposites, where everything is good or bad, pleasant or un-
> pleasant, dry or wet. . . . These contradictions it will find are
> inextricably intertwined (Leboyer, 1975: 41).

The social model of childbirth adheres to a "holistic" view of
woman, encompassing woman as a social, emotional, physical
entity. It views woman in biographical terms, a person with a past
and a future and as part of a larger social structure. This model is
synonymous with the "natural childbirth" philosophy associated
with Dick-Read (1942), Leboyer (1975, 1991), Kitzinger (1978, 1983,
1988) and Odent (1984). According to Wagner (1994: 29) the social
model views life as a solution rather than a problem which is
based on a belief that people can heal themselves and that "medical care should help them in this task, respecting their integrity
and supporting them with the least intervention necessary". With
the social model:

> The person is seen as a kind of ecological system that is not yet
> well understood. This system includes the body, mind and
> spirit, each of which is involved in health and disease. Psycho-
> logical and social factors (such as love and social support or
> lack of them) are emphasised in curing as well as producing
> illness (Wagner, 1994: 29).

The social model was the model previously associated with home
births and domiciliary midwives throughout the western world
(Ehrenreich and English, 1973; Donnison, 1977, 1988; Murphy-
Lawless, 1998a). The medical model of childbirth, according to
Wagner, views life as a problem associated with danger and risk,
which he argues, is "an assumption easily accepted if one's professional career is spent surrounded by pathology, suffering and

death" (1994: 28). Furthermore, Wagner suggests that in the medical model:

> The body is seen as imperfect or even corrupt and health is obtained only with help from the outside. Health is the success of external agents (treatments) over nature in temporarily eliminating disease or other pathological conditions from the body. . . . The best weapons in the struggle against disease and death, according to the medical model, result from the use of the power of science to create the necessary interventions and to determine when and on whom to use them (1994: 28).

The medical model of childbirth, associated with the "active management" philosophy (O'Driscoll et al., 1993), is dominant in maternity units throughout the western world (Stacey, 1988; Oakley, 1993; Tew, 1995; Murphy-Lawless, 1998a). It views woman as a problem to be solved and pregnancy as a pathological state. O'Driscoll et al. (1993: 15) state:

> Before any worthwhile improvement in the conduct of labour could even be contemplated, it was evident that the person ultimately responsible must return to the delivery unit to assume direct responsibility for the welfare of all mothers, not just in theory but also in practice . . . the consultant obstetrician . . . must now become involved directly with the much larger number of perfectly normal women who had hitherto been overlooked at consultant level because they suffered from neither obstetrical complication nor organic disease. Furthermore, it is clear that this commitment must begin at admission and continue until delivery. The consultant, rather than remaining off stage awaiting the occasional summons to perform an emergency operation in a belated attempt to retrieve a situation, which could have been anticipated at a much earlier stage, must seek to prevent such emergencies arising in women who were normal when first admitted to hospital in labour. Ironically, it is in completely normal women that most of the problems of labour arise.

THE MATERNITY PERIOD

Questioning common language raises the question of how "mother" is defined — who is mother, to whom does the term refer? Does it mean the woman who has given birth, is pregnant, in labour, postpartum, the woman whose baby was stillborn, the woman who has had a miscarriage, or the woman who has never given birth but has adopted a baby? All of these women are mothers or potential mothers but for the purpose of this book it is necessary to narrow the focus somewhat. Therefore, the focus of this work is on birth mothers because it is concerned with the physiological aspects of motherhood. The maternity period commences when a woman acknowledges that she is possibly pregnant. Perhaps it is recognised by a combination of factors — that she has had sexual intercourse and that her menstrual period is late or that she feels some physical symptoms usually associated with early pregnancy (Chamberlain, 1995: 37). Any of these factors can mark the beginning of the maternity period for a woman's cognition, whereas for her body the moment of conception is the defining line (Bourne, 1989). Where this period ends is arbitrary as pregnancy and maternity are life-changing experiences and will shape a woman's future in one way or another. However, for the purpose of this book, which cannot span a whole lifetime, the period ends at the infant's first birthday. This is already an important benchmark in social policy as that important statistical measurement and social indicator, the infant mortality rate, is calculated on the basis of infant's death up to the age of one. By this stage, women will have experienced all the policies analysed herein.

LANGUAGE

Language is of vital importance. It is a vital, flowing, constantly changing basis from which to start. Lerner refers to "the power of language to re-name, re-define, re-shape the world . . . the need for re-definition and the inadequacy of terms for describing the female experience, the status of women in society and the various levels of woman's consciousness" (1986: 231). *Life-giving*, for example, is such a positive term. It implies contributing, offering, action, positive participation in something vibrant, alive, promising, energising. An examination of the language associated with the medical and social models of life-giving illuminates the philosophy behind both approaches to childbirth, or more specifically, pregnancy and reproduction. Leboyer, writing in 1975, suggests:

> We must talk to the baby in its own words, the language that precedes words. Are we then to speak in gestures as we would to a foreigner? Of course not. We must go back still further and rediscover the universal language which is simply the language of love. Can this be right for a newborn baby? Yes; we must speak love. We must speak the language of lovers. And what is the universal language of lovers? Not speech. Touch. (Leboyer, 1975: 32).

Leboyer indicates that language sometimes is unnecessary and what is needed is silence:

> This apprenticeship of silence — so indispensable for mothers — is just as important for those who perform the delivery; the obstetricians or midwives. . . . These roaring exhortations upset the mother rather than help her. Lowered voices can relax her, and do far more for her than shouting. . . . People involved in deliveries must learn this new silence, they too must be prepared to receive the child with care and respect (1975: 36).

On the other hand, here is the language used by O'Driscoll et al. writing on the active management of labour, where they negate the importance of language. So, for example, writing on the role of the student midwife, they say:

> The personal nurse is instructed to sit always in front of, and in direct eye contact with, a recumbent mother. . . . Nurses are encouraged to develop close personal relationships with mothers, and to converse with them freely on any subject which holds their interest, thus attracting their attention from

the labour predicament. In our experience, young, properly motivated girls perform this task with remarkable ease when they are made sufficiently conscious of the need, and given the right example by their superiors. . . . The two subjects of conversation which are of abiding interest to a woman in labour are the expected time of delivery and the welfare of the unborn child (O'Driscoll et al., 1993: 103).

The use of language here tends to denigrate both the mother and her attendant, who is referred to as a young girl and as motivated (rather than qualified). In contrast, the words of Leboyer convey an atmosphere of gentleness and respect. The language used by Leboyer has a spiritual element.

TIME

Time is a crucial factor in pregnancy and labour. From the moment a woman is cognisant of her pregnant state, she begins counting dates from the last menstrual period, time of possible ovulation, time of conception, weeks to the expected date of delivery (EDD). When a woman comes into contact with the medical professionals, this is given more substance by taking on written form in charts and medical files. From then on, a woman is given times at which she must reach certain targets, her fundus must be a certain height and her weight must stay within certain parameters. She is given dates and times of future ante-natal appointments, the expected date of delivery and the date at which she will possibly be induced if she has not delivered spontaneously. The active management school uses a chart, a partogram, which allows a woman 12 hours to deliver, measured from the time hospital staff decide the woman is in labour (WHO, 1988). From then on the woman is expected to progress at a certain rate, and if not, then her labour is accelerated. This means that a woman is required to dilate at one centimetre per hour. In the active management school, a woman who does not deliver within 12 hours is generally given a caesarean section. O'Driscoll et al. state categorically:

A formal decision was taken on 1st January 1972 to restrict the
duration of labour to 12 hours. After this date, no provision
was made on the official record for labour to last a longer
time. The result is a well established policy, of which all expectant mothers are fully aware, not to expose anyone to the
stress of labour for more than 12 hours. Meanwhile, in excess
of 150,000 babies have been born and every mother not close
to an easy vaginal delivery after 12 hours has been submitted
to caesarean section (1993: 35).

It must be acknowledged that the majority of women welcome the
promise of a short labour. However, this is a complex subject,
which will be addressed later in this book and has been addressed
elsewhere by numerous writers including MacAdam-O'Connell
(1998) in the Irish context. Murphy-Lawless indicates how:

. . . the focus is on the labour itself, not the woman, and the
overall duration of labour is the central problem, increasing
stress on the woman and risks for the foetus. Time, obstetric
definitions of time rather than the physiological time of the
individual woman, are imposed (1998a: 206).

Time in the social model of childbirth is a different issue. The
woman is recognised as experiencing a very distinct period in her
lifecycle. Pregnancy and birth are acknowledged as a process,
which takes time; all births are different and all women are different. The woman needs time to give birth and the baby needs time
to be born. Leboyer writes:

Patience, or more precisely, the learning of an extreme slowness that borders on immobility. . . . Without this slowness,
success is impossible; without it, we cannot communicate with
a baby. Accepting the slow pace, immersing oneself in it —
this too requires training, as much for the mother as for those
of us who are helping her. Once again, success depends on our
understanding the strange world the baby has inhabited so
far. We must remember that his descent into hell proceeded
centimetre by centimetre, or more slowly still as his movements became more and more constricted . . . his rhythm is so

slow as to be virtually static. Ours is an agitation bordering on frenzy (1975: 37).

Post-natal care is also organised along timescales. Both the social and medical models allocate time in which a woman is expected to recover from childbirth, adjust to her new role and changing body and learn how to nurse her baby. In previous times there existed a lying-in period which enabled a woman to recover, rest, recuperate and learn (Tew, 1995). In recent times women are usually allocated time — time allowed in hospital, time on leave from paid work (these issues are addressed in subsequent chapters). While the social model recognises that the year after birth is a special period in a woman's life (Kitzinger, 1994), the medical model does not allow women the same period of recovery, with a maximum of six weeks' free post-natal care under the Irish Maternity and Infant Care Scheme.

FEAR

Women have learned to fear childbirth, they expect childbirth to be painful, and they fear that pain. Inch claims that:

> . . . perhaps the most potent pain producer is fear. Situations creating fear or anxiety awaken the primitive defence reaction and cause adrenalin and nonadrenalin to be released into the bloodstream (1981: 47).

Feeling fear leads to tension and stress, which in turn lead to even more pain; thus a self-fulfilling prophecy is enacted.

> Who is natural and unselfconscious enough to dare to say I am afraid? Women didn't dare. But their bodies proclaimed it. The bodies of women in labour were a mass of spasms, tensions, frantic heavings, locked muscles. Their bodies sought only to escape, to deny what was taking place; they bore silent witness to their panic and terror. Exorcising this fear has freed women from the agony of childbirth, so that now, at times, it can become almost an ecstasy (Leboyer, 1975: 93).

Sometimes women cannot say they are afraid, or are not heard when they do so, or are not taken seriously:

> As human consciousness is seldom more open to impression than during the momentous hours of labour, a casual approach to just another routine assignment may leave a mother with a burning sense of resentment. Apparently trivial episodes such as curt tone of voice, a blood stained glove, a mindless exposure in the indelicate lithotomy position or a failure to convey the result of pelvic examination, though not seemingly of great consequence in themselves, still portray an often deplorable lack of sensitivity. . . . The steady emotional decline which is a characteristic feature of labour that is not properly supervised, follows an entirely predictable course. . . . The woman becomes progressively withdrawn . . . closes her eyes and buries her head in her pillow . . . to become increasingly restive with contorted features and aimless movements interrupted by frantic outbursts, until eventually a state of panic is reached and self-control is completely lost. . . . A sense of panic is a shattering experience from which the individual may never fully recover. This may lead to recurrent nightmares, permanent revulsion to childbirth with consequent marital disharmony, and a sense of antagonism even towards her own child. Not nearly enough attention is paid to this aspect of trauma in childbirth. Panic should be ranked as one of the most serious complications in obstetrics (O'Driscoll et al., 1993: 93).

While the social model accepts fear as a natural emotion, the medical model views it as an "obstetric complication". O'Driscoll et al. state:

> The disruptive effect of one disorganised and frightened woman in a delivery unit extends far beyond her individual comfort and safety, and there should be no fear in telling her so (1993: 104).

FRAGMENTATION AND SEPARATION (DIVIDE AND CONQUER)

In pregnancy and labour a woman is fragmented. This is a three-fold process. The woman is fragmented from her newborn baby.

Her body is fragmented into parts and she is separated from other women. "Parous women tend to have closed minds on the subject of labour" (O'Driscoll et al., 1993: 79). This is the justification for separating first-time mothers from more experienced women in ante-natal classes:

> Multigravidae are segregated because as a group, their problems are quite different, while, in addition, they are not infrequently prejudiced by past events (O'Driscoll et al., 1993: 79).

Hutter and Williams (1981: 19) refer to the view that "aside from the protection from their own childish nature, pregnant women are seen to need protection from the nature of other women".

Such opinions bring to mind what Oakley has labelled "the subversive power of sisterhood". She illustrates the hostility towards "the existence of a community of alternative purveyors of knowledge about normal motherhood namely other women" (1981a: 101). She argues that advice manuals continually recommend that women should not be encouraged to communicate with each other on the subject of childbirth experiences. This is in stark contrast to Odent's practice at Pithiviers where women meet for ante-natal classes and appointments to partake in a pleasurable sing-a-long session with a pianist to establish a system of social support as well as relaxation.

A woman's body is fragmented by the active management school. The literature talks of the "active uterus". It pays lip service to the emotions. The woman is divided up into a mind and a body but the body is further sub-divided and fragmented. In contrast, in the social school, the woman is viewed in her entirety as a person, as a unit encompassing her unborn child and as part of a larger social fabric, of a social group.

For the nine months preceding delivery, woman and offspring are as one, mother and child are joined. On delivery, at the end of the second stage of labour, this changes. Woman and child become separated. How this is dealt with, managed, controlled and facilitated differs in the social and medical models of childbirth.

> We settle the baby immediately on its mother's stomach. What
> better place could there be? Her stomach has the baby's exact
> shape and dimensions. Swelling a moment before, hollow
> now, the belly seems to lie there waiting, like a nest. And its
> warmth and suppleness as it rises and falls with the rhythm of
> her breathing, its softness, the warmth of its skin, all make it
> the best possible resting place for the child (Leboyer, 1975: 40).

Thus, the inevitable separation of mother and child is dealt with
sensitively. In contrast, the medical model:

> Early adopted the tidier practice of promptly clamping the cord,
> with the disadvantage for the baby of abruptly withdrawing its
> natural support and interrupting the ordered process of transi-
> tion. At the same time it endangered the mother by interfering
> with the physiological process of placental separation and en-
> couraging postpartum haemorrhage. . . . So many hospital-born
> infants have had to share their mothers' drugs that artificial suc-
> tioning of airways has become a routine hospital practice, re-
> gardless of individual need and of the potential damage to the
> infant's respiratory and cardiac systems (Tew, 1995: 184).

Only after all this is done is the baby placed on the mother's
stomach.

CHOICE

> Helping a woman give birth means . . . not preventing her
> from cutting herself off from the outside world. Men have
> never been able to make the interior trip of childbirth and that
> is why many of them can disturb things by their presence
> (Odent, 1984: 140).

The active management school also recognise this "interior trip":

> Nurses are taught that women in labour have a natural ten-
> dency to withdraw from contact with their surroundings and
> turn inwards on themselves, and that this inclination to intro-
> spection is exaggerated greatly by analgesic drugs. They are
> forewarned about the woman who closes her eyes, buries her
> face in the pillow and continues to complain even between

contractions. They know that these are the signs which indicate that the thread of personal contact is being eroded and that, once broken, it will be very difficult to mend. They are acutely sensitive to the fact that the woman who turns her back is passing a devastating judgement on the quality of the nursing care (O'Driscoll et al., 1993: 102).

Choice involves freedom, opportunity to participate, to decide to disclaim, repudiate, accept, all options often denied women in labour. Michel Odent recognises that:

Everyone who has tried to understand what makes childbirth easier, less painful, shorter and thus less dangerous is agreed. They all emphasize the importance of a familiar and feminine environment. They know that the presence of a doctor is often inhibiting. They know that when you have to go from one place to another during labour it can often disturb things. And they know how important are semi-darkness, silence, warmth and freedom of posture (1984: 132).

"Right to choose" is a term very explicitly associated with women's control over their own reproduction, but it is one rarely associated with a woman's right to choose how, where and when she chooses to give birth. This is a concept that has been removed from women's experience of childbirth.

When roughly four-fifths of the population of the western world live less than 20 minutes from a hospital equipped to do caesareans; when even ambulances for dogs have the equipment needed to do emergency surgery, there can be no rational basis for the discredit accorded to home birth. The discredit is based on a lack of will. The subtlest way to discredit home birth is to make it as dangerous as possible. It is made dangerous partly by creating an atmosphere of guilt. When a woman dares to think of having a home birth, the first thing she is asked is what she would do if there were complications (Odent, 1984: 133).

The medical model refers to women using their own initiative:

Uniquely, an expectant mother admits herself to a maternity hospital with the result that she tends to dictate her own treatment. This method of procedure, which leaves the initiative in the hands of "patients", has no parallel in other branches of medicine . . . the most surprising feature is not that mothers are sometimes wrong but that they are usually right. . . . The general assumption is that no such problem exists because women are naturally endowed with an unerring instinct that enables them to make a correct decision in these matters (O'Driscoll et al., 1993: 36).

CONTROL

It appears that the only decision a pregnant woman makes is to visit the doctor in the first place; after that the whole matter is taken out of her hands (Oakley, 1981a: 80).

Control is a very significant concept. Control, with all its connotations — domination, power, superiority, authority, suppression, oppression, powerlessness — is the essence of patriarchy. The patriarchal control of childbirth has been increasing over the last century. Rich refers to "the rapidly increasing complexity of systems and the training of elite males who will decide how and for what technology is to be used" (Rich, 1980: 264). Personal communication with the Institute of Obstetrics and Gynaecology in 2002 confirmed that at present about 60 per cent of those in training in Dublin, Galway, Cork and Limerick are women while ten years ago the figure was only five per cent. At present women consultants account for about 20 per cent of those in Irish maternity units. Thus, while there has been an increase in the number of women working at higher levels in obstetrics, men still dominate; at the same time, the predominantly female midwifery profession appears to be more disempowered than ever. This power is the ultimate control by men over women in the most intimate physiological process. Sometimes there is an illusion of shared control:

No examination is undertaken on a woman without her direct involvement and in deference to her before, during and after

the event. . . . Regular pelvic examination should be mandatory
after each of the first three hours (O'Driscoll et al., 1993: 46).

The woman does not decide when to leave hospital. In the case of
a "false labour":

> . . . she is not allowed home . . . until, she is formally dis-
> charged on the following day. This precaution eliminates the
> possible embarrassment of giving birth in transit (O'Driscoll et
> al., 1993: 42).

As childbirth has moved from the private to the public domain, as
gradually childbirth has been taken over by the male medical profession, control by women of their own bodies and pregnancies
and labours has been lost. As Rich suggests:

> It is increasingly clear that medical technology has . . . become
> a means of alienating women from the act of giving birth,
> hence from their own bodies, their own creative powers, and
> of keeping birth itself so far as possible in male control. It has
> also become a major industry (1980: 268).

DIGNITY

> The voices of a few women raised in warning cannot be heard
> over the humming and throbbing of our machines, which is
> probably just as well, for if we succeed in crushing all pride
> and dignity out of child bearing, the population explosion will
> take care of itself (Greer, 1985: 30).

Women constantly refer to being made to feel exposed, embarrassed, violated in the labour ward (*Mother and Child Conference*,
1996; *Changing Childbirth Now* workshop — facilitated by this author — 1997). For many women, this process begins on entering the
maternity unit when their clothes are taken from them. Others refer
to the presence of unwanted and unnecessary persons in the delivery ward, while others refer to the postpartum period when they
are not allowed to avail of bath and shower facilities, sometimes
due to lack of personnel, often due to time of day or night, and are

left feeling dirty. Others refer to the lack of hygiene in the labour ward while others refer to the way in which they are addressed by hospital personnel (Kennedy and Murphy-Lawless, 2002).

Sometimes women feel that they are not listened to, and that their wishes are not respected. There appears to be an underlying belief in obstetrics that a woman is not in tune with her own reproductive system and may have problems in language comprehension. Looking at the active management school, there apparently is a lack of respect for the mother:

> Naturally, whenever a woman's presumptive diagnosis of labour is not accepted by staff she deserves an adequate explanation couched in simple language which she can understand (O'Driscoll et al., 1993: 37).

Odent (1984: 138) asks why it is that for thousands of years women in labour have always hidden away from men's eyes while they give birth. "Privacy is indeed the key word in understanding the needs of a woman giving birth, privacy is what you feel when there is no social control" (Odent, 1984: 139). O'Driscoll et al. espouse a theory why this might be so:

> Some women suffer from intractable nausea and vomiting, sufficient to turn childbirth into a miserable experience. Some become profoundly depressed, introspective, and so overwhelmed with self-pity that they lapse eventually into a state of stupor, from which they are roused only by contractions, to make aimless protests and demand more and more drugs, until the original position is compounded and a vicious circle is established (O'Driscoll et al., 1993: 82).

COST

There is a cost associated with childbirth. The active management school would appear to view this cost in terms of hospital resources:

> The delivery unit constitutes the bottleneck in a maternity unit through which all consumers must pass . . . it is not possible to

plan maternity hospital accommodation, or to allocate professional staff on a rational basis, unless the number of consumer
hours to be serviced can be calculated in advance. Here is a
prime example of the application of principles of cost effi-
ciency in contemporary medical planning, where good medicine and sound economics are seen to complement each other.
Nowhere is this seen to better advantage than in a modern, ef-
ficient intensive care delivery unit (O'Driscoll et al, 1993: 34).

To the mother there is often the cost of lost innocence, confidence,
dignity and shattered dreams. A woman can be robbed of her confidence, self-belief and the joy of an empowering, fulfilling birth
experience. As Inch indicates, childbirth for women "is an event
which will colour and shape the remainder of their lives . . . many
emerge from the experience much sadder and wiser" (1981: 1).
She can be robbed of privacy, dignity and respect. The child can
be robbed of a pleasant passage. There are real financial costs too
associated with the birth of a child, particularly a first child, as
will be explored in later chapters.

POWER

Inch indicates that women's feelings can be disregarded in a hospital setting because "power relationships between givers and receivers of care, both in pregnancy and labour, are often unequal"
(1981: 70). This, she argues, is due to the size and complexity of
hospitals, which are bureaucratic and hierarchically organised institutions. She argues that status and role can dominate "the more
personal and spontaneous factors that characterise relationships
in the less public spheres of life" (1981: 70). In contrast, the social
model stresses that mothers often describe childbirth as empowering, while others stress that what they have experienced is an
overwhelming feeling of powerlessness (O'Connor, 1992, 1995,
1998). Kitzinger claims that during labour "women learn that it
pays to be passive" (1983: 20), indicating that women who are as-
sertive or protest are frowned upon in the medical model of
childbirth. As O'Driscoll et al. remind us:

... nurses are not expected to submit themselves to the sometimes outrageous conduct of perfectly healthy women who
cannot be persuaded to cross a narrow corridor from an ante-
natal clinic. Such women must learn to behave with dignity
and purpose during the most important event of their lives.
Nor should nurses be held responsible for the degrading
scenes which occasionally result from failure of a woman to
fulfil her part of the compact (1993: 104).

Looking to education as the answer, O'Driscoll et al. claim, "the
authors never cease to be impressed by the ability of the average
woman to assimilate the essential facts about labour when these
are properly presented" (1993: 105).

PLACE

The social model refers to the importance of place, often stressing
the advantages of women choosing to give birth in the familiar
surroundings of one's own home. In the early decades of this century women often favoured hospital-based childbirth as they then
had a ten-day lying-in period (Tew, 1995) which gave the women,
often from poorer households, a chance to rest, recuperate and
escape from the arduous domestic chores which they had to en-
dure. This may still be the case for many women. However, hospitals nowadays tend to be bigger, and as a result noisier, busier
and less restful places to be and the stay there limited to one or
two days after delivery. As Kitzinger indicates:

Women often said that they had too little rest in hospital and
some discharged themselves so that they could get more rest
at home. A few mentioned that they took some time recovering from the rush and bustle of hospital. But, and this is significant, it was hardly ever rest from the baby that they
wanted, but rest from hospital routines which meant that
sleep or cuddling or feeding-time with the baby was interrupted or, in a few hospitals, that the husband's or other children's visits were rushed (1983: 138).

The hospitalisation of childbirth involves ritual:

Western culture has surrounded birth by hospital routines, many of which are ceremonial procedures functioning to turn a woman into a patient, and then processing her through the system to emerge at the other end as a mother and a new baby. These rites serve to reinforce the power of the hospital as an institution, and that of the professionals who bear responsibility for the outcome of birth, as against the mothers, who are merely the objects of their care (Kitzinger, 1983: 30).

The place where the woman gives birth has implications also for financial costs of the exercise. The 2001 evaluation of the National Maternity Hospital Community Midwifery Service indicates that the cost of implementing the project amounted to an average cost of delivery of €2,087.88, while the average cost of delivery in the National Maternity Hospital was €2,820.67 (Women's Health Unit, 2001) Nowadays there is a real pressure on hospitals to limit financial costs. Referring to the cost associated with hospital births, O'Driscoll et al. indicate that:

. . . the new-found ability to limit the duration of stay and therefore quantify the total number of consumer hours to be serviced, has transformed the previously haphazard approach to planning in this area (1993: 114).

Referring to place of birth when that place is home, Kitzinger indicates:

When a woman gives birth at home the territory is controlled by the family and the doctor and the midwives are guests. In birth at home the mother is the central actor in the drama and everyone else is there to serve her and her baby. There is no management system by which she is processed or with which she has to cope (1983: 102).

HEALTH AND SAFETY

The debate around safety in childbirth is presented in detail in Chapter Six of this book. The social model stresses that "birth is a major and unique event that is remembered for a lifetime; and it is

not just a matter of a healthy mother and child" (Inch, 1981: 69).
On the other hand, the medical model stresses:

> All kinds of obstetric intervention to ensure that the pattern of
> labour relates to a norm, devised by obstetricians, of how la-
> bour should be. The intervention is planned to prevent rather
> than to cure. It is based on the concept that birth is always po-
> tentially hazardous and should be conducted in an intensive
> care situation (Kitzinger, 1983: 45).

Adhering to a social model of childbirth, Inch states that "there is
a great deal more to being alive than simply not being dead"
(1989: 66). Referring to morbidity, Inch states:

> There are other sorts of morbidity which are so common that
> the mother may be regarded as "well" by the traditional crite-
> ria for successful obstetric management; episiotomy, for ex-
> ample. It is also difficult to see how the objective world of
> obstetric concern would classify the psychological damage to a
> woman, which can have repercussions beyond the immediate
> post-natal period (1989: 66).

Having presented the social and medical models of childbirth
through the lens of the concepts of language, time, fear, fragmentation, choice, control, dignity, cost, power, place, health and
safety, this book now proceeds to explore Irish mothers' experiences as they progress through the maternity period in the Irish
maternity care system. The focus is broadened from the physiological to the three-dimensional model of motherhood.

Chapter Three

THE HISTORICAL DIMENSION

This chapter introduces the historical issues, ideologies and events that have shaped social policies which are directly relevant to women as they experience pregnancy and the first year of maternity in Ireland. The chapter begins with an introduction to the emerging welfare state before going on to look chronologically at issues and events that have influenced the development of Irish health, welfare and labour market policies.

Looking at Ireland as a conservative/corporatist-type state highlights the institutional and organisational aspects of welfare provision. Conservative/corporatist regimes are characterised by strong church influence, status-differentiated social insurance, underdevelopment of day care and other family services, the principle of subsidiarity is strong and political coalition-building prevails (Esping Andersen, 1990; Breen et al., 1990; McLaughlin, 1993). To quote Siim, "the state today has come to play a crucial role in determining the position of women as workers, mothers and citizens . . . the state has nowhere been neutral to women" (1988: 160). Reference here to welfare states means not only the provision of welfare in the traditional sense of health, housing, education, income maintenance and the personal social services, but also the broader political economy in which the state is located together with its underlying ideologies. As Wilson states, "the welfare state is made up of both the welfare policies and the ideologies in which they come wrapped" (1977: 12). Ireland typifies a "mixed economy of welfare" with welfare provision coming from a variety of sources: the statutory, private, informal and voluntary sectors (Fanning, 1999).

Social policy does not emerge from a vacuum. Rather, it emerges or is etched out of the historical context and social structures of the society in which it develops, with the help or hindrance of the leading actors of the time. Looking at Irish social policies which have particular significance for women in Ireland as they experience pregnancy and maternity, it is necessary to tease out who and what were these critical influences. This chapter begins by looking at some of the major ideological influences prevalent in Ireland in the decades following Independence. Secondly, it outlines the main legislative and policy developments in Ireland relevant to pregnant women and mothers of young children since the Irish welfare state began to emerge.

FOUNDATIONS

The historical development of social policies in Ireland has been widely analysed (Maguire, 1986; Burke, 1987; Powell, 1992; Barrington, 1987). The newly independent state inherited the beginnings of a welfare state from the British administration whose foundations were laid with the introduction of the Poor Relief (Ireland) Act of 1838. That Act established the workhouse system and the Amendment Act of 1847 provided outdoor relief. The Medical Charities Act of 1851 set up a national dispensary medical service and the Public Health (Ireland) Act 1878 marked the beginning of a public health system. A national system of primary education had been established in 1831. The 1911 National Insurance Act introduced social insurance to Ireland while the controversy surrounding the medical section of that Act demonstrated the readiness of the Irish Catholic hierarchy to get involved in social policy issues (Barrington, 1987: 64).

Social policies and legislation of particular relevance to mothers and children in the period 1900–1921 included the 1907 Notification of Births Act, which Barrington says, "to the extent it applied in Ireland, was a first step in the direction of public provision for mothers and children" (1987: 76). This Act, which was permissive, allowed the urban sanitary authorities to notify the medical officer of each district of birth (official registration of births was compulsory since 1863) and to organise health visiting for mothers and babies. Barrington highlights how the permissive nature of this Act ensured that by 1915 it was adopted only in Dublin and Belfast and "only in Dublin were special 'sanitary officers' appointed for the purpose of visiting and advising mothers" (1987: 76). The legislation was tightened in that year when powers were given to sanitary authorities in urban areas to provide for the needs of mothers and children. The Local Government Board was encouraged to develop schemes aimed at protecting the health of mothers and children. Again, this legislation was permissive and thus limited in its application. Barrington (1987: 77) highlights the possible scope of this scheme which empowered local authorities to appoint health visitors to provide advice and services for expecting and nursing mothers at home, as well as services for infants and the services of a midwife or doctor, and hospital treatment at confinement and food for women and children based on evidence of need.

Robins (2000) indicates that the earliest formalised midwifery education dates back to 1773 in the Rotunda, then known as the Dublin Lying-In Hospital, with the Coombe Lying-in Hospital introducing training in 1836 and the Royal College of Physicians of Ireland and Sir Patrick Dun's in 1868. Scanlan (1991: 92) indicates the importance of midwifery legislation in Ireland at the turn of this century. The 1902 Midwives Act, which was intended to better midwifery training and to regulate midwifery practice, did not extend to Ireland. However, it did provide for the recognition of midwives trained by the Royal College of Physicians, the Coombe and the Rotunda Hospitals.

The Midwives (Ireland) Act, which was passed in 1917, prohibited unqualified women from practising as midwives and established a Midwives Board. Scanlan summarises the objectives of the 1917 Act as: confining midwifery practice to qualified, registered midwives; the establishment of a Central Midwives Board; and the designation of powers and responsibilities of the local supervising authorities concerning the practice of midwifery. The Act, according to Scanlan (1991: 94), came into effect almost im-

mediately with regard to women practising midwifery without
being recognised by law. The institutions recognised in regard to
training of midwives were the Coombe, the Rotunda and the National Maternity Hospitals, the Incorporated Maternity Hospital
in Belfast, the Cork Lying-In Hospitals and the Bedford Row
Hospital in Limerick. During the first six months of its existence,
the Board granted 1,120 applications for enrolment as midwives.

In 1918, the Local Government Board stated it would make
substantial contributions towards salaries for midwives, health
visitors and nurses engaged in maternal and child welfare. It also
provided assistance towards convalescent care, and contributions
towards voluntary organisations engaged in maternal and child
health schemes. This, Barrington (1987) claims, seems to have
been an effective measure. Scanlan draws attention to two important measures introduced during the 1920s. First of all, the authority was granted to midwives, when in practice under a
supervising authority, to possess and administer opium-
containing preparations. Secondly, the required period of midwifery training was increased from six months for trained nurses
to one year for those without nursing training.

Regarding income maintenance, the 1911 National Insurance
Act ensured that maternity benefit of 30 shillings was paid to an
insured worker or to the wife of an insured male worker as a
once-off payment to meet the extra costs associated with childbirth (the subsequent development of such payments is addressed
in Chapter Eleven). Barrington states that "this relatively large
sum was to pay for the extra expenses of childbirth and to encourage working mothers to remain at home with the child in the
early months" (1987: 76), and indicates that in 1915 benefit was
paid in respect of just less than half the births in the country. This
was to change radically in the remainder of the century, as will be
demonstrated later on in this book.

The emergence of the new state brought with it a series of legislative and constitutional changes which have since shaped the
nature and scope of pregnancy and maternity policies in Ireland:

Throughout the period 1922–1961 a series of legislative measures were enacted by the governments of the day, which had
the purpose of clearly delineating the place of women in society. These measures both reflected and helped to shape the social norms of Ireland during the period (Conroy Jackson, 1993:
74).

FROM INDEPENDENCE TO THE EMERGENCY

The newly independent Ireland that emerged in 1922 after a very
violent and turbulent decade as a result of the struggle for independence was characterised at first by civil war, by widespread
poverty both rural and urban, the prevalence of TB, a high incidence of unemployment, poor infrastructure and a concern with
controlling law and order (Lyons, 1973; O'Hagan, 1975; Tierney,
1978; Fanning, 1983; Barrington, 1987). Fanning refers to how the
1920s in Ireland were plagued by the financial costs of the civil
war (1983: 39). In the year from 1923 to 1924, 30 per cent of all national expenditure was on defence and a further 7 per cent on
compensation for loss of property and personal injury, and this
pattern continued to a lesser extent throughout the 1920s. Manning (1987: 13) argues that the Cumann na nGaedhael government angered teachers, police, civil servants and old age
pensioners through threatening to cut their pay: "during its 10
years in power politics were neither radical or revolutionary"
(Manning, 1987: 5). Ó Gráda states that "the economic policies
pursued by those who ruled the Irish free state between 1922 and
1932 made virtues of continuity and caution" (1997: 4). Under
Cumann na nGaedheal (1922–1932), the population decline continued, as did the emigration and unemployment that had esca-
lated with the great famine in the middle of the nineteenth
century (Ó Gráda, 1997).

On achieving independence, Ireland was an underdeveloped,
isolated and traditional society (Lee, 1989). The 1926 Census re-
vealed that 53 per cent of the productive workforce was employed
in agriculture. Fanning refers to the underdevelopment of industry in Ireland where "only 8 per cent of the population were wage

earners of 16 years and upwards in industry and commerce" (1983: 76). In 1926, out of 329,000 women at work, six out of ten were in either farming or domestic service while one-tenth worked in industry (Daly, 1978: 71). Ireland existed economically on the periphery of Britain. Fanning (1983) refers to the obstacles to industrial development as including a home market too small to enable home producers to compete with imports, little or no export trade to enable large factories succeed and a lack of factors which would attract foreign investment. O'Hagan indicates that the new government was:

> Not well equipped in terms of economic expertise, its intellectual members being predominantly literary men rather than economists, and it depended for economic guidance on conservatively minded advisers, who advocated caution in regard to any moves that would separate the new state economically from the United Kingdom (1975: 7).

Fanning refers to how difficult it was to "expunge Victorian mentalities" (1983: *vii*). The historian Mary Daly (1995: 100) reminds us that "the primacy given to political change and to the culture and ideology of the independent Irish state tends to detract attention from the influence of economic factors on the lives of Irish women". Daly (1995: 101) indicates that by the time of the first population census in the Irish Free State taken in 1926, Irish women, both married and single, had a low labour market participation rate with a high concentration in both agriculture and domestic service and a high proportion employed within the family economy. Daly (1995) indicates that 24 per cent of women in the 45–54 age group were single in 1926, at a time when unemployment was very high among single women. Declining female employment in manufacturing reflected the collapse of the domestic textile industry. Women were a majority of emigrants until the beginning of the Second World War. For women in employment in 1926, 60 per cent of jobs were in agriculture and domestic service and "the family economy continued to loom large in Irish female employment" (1995: 105). They were also employed in family shops and businesses. Daly refers to the establishment of the new Irish civil service as a provider of employment opportunities for women: "the number of established female civil servants increased by 140 per cent during the first ten years of the Irish Free State from 940 to 2,260" (Daly, 1995: 107).

In urban Ireland in 1926, 120 out of 1,000 babies died in their first year of life. In 1928/29 there were over 3,500 deaths from TB, and the Department of Health estimated that for each death there existed eight sufferers (Barrington, 1987: 105). In this harsh social and economic environment, Irish women as mothers had to cope with the day-to-day realities of making ends meet and struggling against poverty. Guilbride (1996) refers to the "underfed, anaemic mothers of large families working on farms or in low paid menial jobs in the cities, who were . . . respectable married women" and asks "if their economic and social status was so low, what hope was there for those mothers who were branded with the stigma of an illegitimate child" (1996: 88).

The 1927 *Report of the Commission on the Relief of the Sick and Destitute Poor including the Insane Poor* differentiated between different groups of mothers, namely married mothers, widows and unmarried mothers divided into two groups, those "who may be considered amenable to reform" and those "regarded as less hopeful cases" (1927: 68). In this latter category, they included married mothers who had children "not the offspring of their husbands". The Report referred to "first offenders" and those "who had fallen more than once" (1927: 69). The recommendations of this report included:

> If an unmarried woman who applies for relief during pregnancy or after giving birth to a child is willing, when applying for assistance, to undertake to remain for a period not exceeding one year there should be power to retain her for that period, in the case of a first admission. In the case of admission for a second time, there should be power to retain her for a period of two years. On third or subsequent admissions the Board should have power to retain for such a period as they think fit having considered on recommendation of the Supe-

rior or Matron of the Home. All cases whose maximum period
of residence is indeterminate should be reviewed annually
(1927: 69).

Furthermore, this report indicated that such mothers should take
part in useful employment. Alarmingly, this report recommended
that:

> We have come to the conclusion that no woman should be dis-
> charged until she has satisfied the Board of Health that she will
> be able to provide for her child or children, either by way of pay-
> ing wholly or partially for maintenance in the home or boarding
> out with respectable people approved by the Health Board. Dis-
> cretion might be allowed . . . to allow the woman to take her dis-
> charge without taking her child or children (1927: 69).

Referring specifically to the offspring of unmarried mothers, the
1927 report refers to the high mortality rate of these young infants,
with one out of four not surviving the first year of life. The high
death rate was explained not as due to economic difficulties but
because "the illegitimate child, being the proof of the mother's
shame is, in most cases, sought to be hidden at all costs" (1927: 69).

Women as wives and mothers were obliged to stay at home by
restrictive employment practices such as the "marriage bar" of 1929
and the "baby bar", and by welfare policies which institutionalised
women's dependency status (Conroy Jackson, 1993). Throughout
the 1920s, a series of legislative measures particularly relevant to
women's lives were introduced. These included the 1924/1927 Juries Act which made it almost impossible for women to serve on
juries (Valiulis, 1997; Robinson, 1978) and the 1929 Censorship of
Publications Act, which denied women access to contraceptive information.

Lee indicates that post-independence Ireland was "a relatively
modernised society" (1989: 69) and that the standard of living here
was similar to the rest of Europe, that was, two-thirds that of Britain. However, he states, "the manner in which Ireland achieved
this average was unique . . . and potentially debilitating" (1989:
70). In 1931, there were 45,000 farms of less than one acre, run on a

subsistence level and 58 per cent of all farms were between one and 30 acres. Lee indicates that "rural Ireland not only controlled numbers in a clinical manner but also effectively controlled the social structure" (1989: 71). Only 19 per cent of those working on farms were paid employees (Tierney, 1978: 200).

However, Lee (1989: 77) claims that the Free State inherited relatively strong economic, educational, social and political infrastructures. It had a complex and diversified occupational structure:

> A callously efficient socialisation process postponed marriage and effectively denied the right to a family to a higher proportion of the population than in any other European state, by the simple device of parents disinheriting a high proportion of potential grooms and brides among their children. The dispossessed were reconciled to their fate by emigration, high emigration continued to channel the potential resentment of the disinherited out of the country (Lee, 1989: 71).

THE THIRTIES

As the new decade began, 8.5 per cent of school children inspected in 1931 were suffering from malnutrition and "the majority of children were verminous" (Barrington, 1987: 103). As a result of these inspections, 26,000 children were treated. Ireland's free trade policies continued up until 1932 when the anti-treaty party led by de Valera, now called Fianna Fáil, came to power for the first time since Independence. Fianna Fáil was characterised by a strong nationalist philosophy eager to attain economic and cultural sovereignty. Protectionist policies were introduced, reflecting a *sinn féin* ("we ourselves") philosophy, manifested in high tariffs, national self-sufficiency (aiming to end the country's economic dependence on Britain) and nationalist orthodoxy, culminating in a new Constitution in 1937. The protectionist policies increased Ireland's isolation. Fianna Fáil decided not to pay the land annuities, withholding them from July 1932. The British Government retaliated by imposing tariffs on Irish agricultural and cattle exports. The Irish Government in return introduced tariffs on certain British imports including coal, machinery and cement. Tierney (1978: 201) describes the economic war which lasted until 1938 as "disastrous for Ireland", indicating that it caused a serious depression of agriculture, a considerable reduction in the income of farmers, a huge decrease in the income of agricultural labourers, the almost complete destruction of the cattle industry and an increase in unemployment. The period was marked by a very high level of emigration from Ireland to Britain and the United States. Emigration was particularly high amongst Irish women (Jackson, 1987b).

The 1930s witnessed the passing of legislation which was particularly restrictive for Irish women. The Dance Halls Act of 1935 ushered in restrictions on social activities and in the same year the Criminal Law Amendment Act banned the importation and sale of contraceptives. In the following year, the Conditions of Employment Act placed restrictions on women's access to paid employment.

The Constitution

The 1937 Constitution clarifies the position of the family in Irish life. McLaughlin writes:

> Women's fears that the state and the Catholic church were determined to push through enforced domestication were confirmed when De Valera unveiled the 1937 constitution . . . it gave formal recognition to the "holy trinity" of the family, the Church and the nation and outlined a series of social policy principles which were intended to re-establish and reinforce traditional gender relations by removing women from public life (1993: 210).

The 1937 Constitution grew out of a period when there was a "moral crisis" in Catholic Ireland. An increase in illegitimacy rates had led to a public outcry and the closure of many dance halls, strict legislation on censorship, alcohol and such like measures (Whyte, 1980). The Government began to take an interest in social education with the introduction of policies geared towards controlling young people and promoting very traditional values

(Kennedy, 1984). The Constitution was seen as a perfect opportunity to promote Catholic social teaching and to control the citizens of Ireland, and in particular women, and to reverse the 1922–1936 Constitution.

In the 1937 Constitution, the "family" was given a special status in Irish society. De Valera's ideology, as represented in the constitutional articles on women and the family, undoubtedly echoed Papal teaching: "let women be subject to their husbands as to the Lord, because the husband is the head of the wife, as Christ is the head of the Church" (*Castii Conubii*, 1930: 13). Mary Robinson indicates how the English text uses the term *woman* as opposed to the Irish *Bean an Tí*, which she says, "is at least a fair inference that even in 1937 it was intended to refer to the married woman" (1978: 61).

Article 41.

1.1 The State recognises the Family as the natural primary unit group of Society, and as a moral institution possessing inalienable and imprescriptible rights, antecedent and superior to all positive law.

1.2 The State, therefore, guarantees to protect the Family in its Constitution and authority, as the necessary basis of social order and as indispensable to the welfare of the Nation and the State.

This status of the family hinged to a large extent on "woman" or "mother" who was also endowed with a particularly "favoured" status, which she was expected to live out within the home.

Article 41.2

1. In particular, the State recognises that by her life within the home, woman gives to the State a support without which the common good cannot be achieved.

2. The State shall, therefore, endeavour to ensure that mothers shall not be obliged by economic necessity to engage in labour to the neglect of their duties in the home.

These articles find resonance in Rich, who states that there "has been a basic contradiction throughout patriarchy; between the laws and sanctions designed to keep women essentially powerless and the attribution to mothers of almost superhuman power (of control, of influence, of life-support)" (1977: 263–264).

There were significant developments in social legislation during the 1930s, which were in line with the values propounded in the 1937 Constitution, shaped by de Valera and Catholic social teaching. As Barrington puts it, "and brooding behind every aspect of Irish life is the church" (1987: 2). For a long period Irish life was regarded as synonymous with Catholicism, whose values were incorporated into the Irish Constitution of 1937. Breen et al. refer to that Constitution as "an amalgam of Catholic moral principles, nationalist aspirations, and American precedents, the latter being evident in its liberal ideas on human rights" (1990: 29). Fanning states:

> What happened was that the church in independent Ireland swiftly adopted . . . support for government and opposition to revolution. . . . If the Catholic hierarchy was no longer disposed to question the authority of the state, neither were the rulers of the infant state disposed to question the authority of the Catholic Church, not at least in such matters as health, education and sexual morality where the church was deemed to have a special competence (1983: 53).

O'Dowd attempts to explore why "political ideology and religion contributed to the contraction of women's public and political role in the period between the Treaty and the outbreak of world war" (1986: 40). He refers to three factors — firstly, the international context; secondly, images of women promulgated in Ireland within Church and State; and thirdly, evidence from census material — as an indication of the broader cultural assumptions about women's role. He refers to "sustained attempts to confine women to the private or familial sphere in the period under study" (1987: 50). O'Dowd refers to the male-dominated institutions of church and state which have "either ignored or marginalised the social role of women, or, alternatively, consigned women to a servicing and largely invisible role outside 'history' and 'politics'" (1987: 5). At the same time, O'Dowd acknowledges that "conservatism, national chauvinism and isolationism in the 1937 Constitution, were by no means an Irish monopoly" (1987: 6), referring to Stalinist pro-natalist and pro-family policy. O'Dowd states that, in the light of high unemployment, the labour movement was "highly ambivalent on the question of female, especially unmarried, female participation in the labour force" (1987: 7). According to O'Dowd, the success of the Catholic Church was due in part to "the lack of ideological competitors" (1987: 12). Secondly, "the Catholic Church had a large body of well-educated professionals, the clergy, at their disposal, and a well-established institutional structure including publications and an accepted means of communication via the pulpit, the open air meeting and household visitation (1987: 13).

Mahon points to the necessity of looking to the Constitution in analysing Irish women's peculiar position. She states that "the 1937 Constitution endorses a patriarchal system in which the male is the breadwinner and the woman is confined to the domestic sphere" (1987: 56). This male breadwinner model (Lewis, 1993) was reinforced by the determination of both Church and State to adhere to the principle of subsidiarity. MacCurtain questions:

> After the Civil War . . . a generation of sorrowful and purposeful women turned their faces forward to reconstruction of their shattered country. . . . Irish women were free in the areas they had struggled for, why then were they content to remain subordinate in a society they had helped to create? (1978: 56).

The reasons were many, political, cultural and social, but with one strong thread running throughout: the Church and State united to define women's position, which was very much in the home and as wife and mother. The Catholic Church was particularly strong in the newly independent Ireland. As Whyte indicates, "caught between the anarchy of traditional capitalism on the one hand and the totalitarianism of the left on the other, Catholics believed that the Pope had shown them a way out" (1980: 68). Whyte (1980: 3) illustrates the strength of Catholicism in the decades which coincide with the development of the Irish Welfare State as follows: "since independence, the proportion of Roman Catholics has risen with every count; 92.6 per cent in 1926, 93.4 per cent in 1936, 94.3 per cent in 1946 and 94.9 per cent in 1961". It is necessary to examine what other factors led Irish political leaders down the path which earned them the title of "the most conservative revolutionaries in history". Ward (1983) indicates however that such conservatism did not go unchallenged by the women of Ireland.

Patriarchy

Walby defines patriarchy as "a system of social structures and practices in which men dominate, oppress and exploit women" (1990: 20). In the period under study in this chapter, the Church most definitely intervened explicitly and forcefully in State affairs. Breen et al. (1990) highlight the extent of patriarchy in Ireland, which they regard as very much linked to Catholicism and to the familial character of Irish society. Patriarchy was a strong feature in regulating the economy. Fathers' decisions and influence over inheritance in turn affected decisions and the economic freedom to marry, which was not easy for a couple in a society where regular and frequent procreation was the norm. Lee highlights how "social values prevented a higher proportion of women from becoming mothers than in any other European country" (1989: 158). In a country where a couple married at a later age than their European contemporaries, they still boasted higher fertility rates because of the absence of birth control (Solomons, 1992). Ireland still has the highest fertility rate in the European Union.

Guilbride claims that "the social and moral ideology of any state is invariably determined by the economic conditions which underpin the ideology (1996: 85). Guilbride explores the history of infanticide from the inception of the State up to the 1950s. She indicates that:

> . . . a salient point here is that motherhood was dependent on marriage. Economic factors prevented women from marrying, and social values prevented women from becoming mothers but they did not prevent them from becoming pregnant (1996: 87).

Regarding options available to women who conceived outside of marriage, Jackson (1987a) outlines the reality of the situation for women in Ireland following legislative measures of the 1930s and 1940s. She refers to how the medicalisation of reproduction combined with the subordination of women's reproduction and sexuality in the legal, social and cultural instances drove the demand for abortion underground in Ireland. She claims that from 1922 to 1965, backstreet abortion was practised in Ireland, as can be seen from the number of judicial proceedings prior to 1967 when abortion laws in Britain were relaxed. Jackson indicates that backstreet abortion was engaged in by women of different social classes throughout the country and particularly during the Second World War when travel to England was restricted to those going for business purposes or for designated seasonal work.

Guilbride's research indicates that one way of dealing with an extramarital pregnancy in Ireland was infanticide and, interestingly, in the cases examined by her almost all the women were classed as poor or destitute, more than half were employed as farm labourers while more than a third were domestic servants. Infanticide soared in Ireland during the 1940s after the passage of the 1935 Criminal Law (Amendment) Act that banned contraception and the Emergency Powers Act which prohibited travel from Ireland during the Second World War. Guilbride concludes that "infanticide in this state and throughout most of this century at least, has been constantly linked to illegitimacy and economic deprivation" (1996: 85).

For those women who obeyed the prescribed rules of Church and State and gave birth to legitimate children, the power of the Church still loomed over their shoulders. Johnston, recalling life in inner city Dublin in the 1930s and 1940s, recounts:

> As soon as the mother got to her feet after the birth, her first
> duty was to be churched. This was a thanksgiving service after
> safe birth and although in theory it was voluntary, all the
> mothers felt . . . that it was compulsory, and in a sense it was
> because social pressure forced women to go . . . women had to
> be cleansed after giving birth, implying in some way that it
> was dirty (Johnston, 1985: 71).

Johnston goes on to describe this ceremony:

> The ceremony required that the woman kneel at the entrance
> of the church holding a lighted candle. The priest would then
> touch her with the end of his stole and introduce her into the
> church with prayers and holy water (1985: 71).

This humiliating act had a very significant place in Irish society
and was an important force in relating female sexuality, conception and childbirth to shame and sin.

The 1937 Constitution was formulated in the wake of the publication of the 1931 Papal encyclical *Quadragesimo Anno* (1931)
which Esping-Andersen refers to when he claims that "Corporatist welfare became the dogma of the Catholic Church and was
actively espoused in the two major papal encyclicals" (1990: 40).
Referring to the 1931 encyclical he remarks, "the corporatist element was especially strong and was in line with current Fascist
ideology" (1990: 40). This ideology was not unique to Ireland but
was also favoured by Germany, Austria and Spain. As Esping-
Andersen indicates, "the ulterior motives were social integration,
the preservation of authority, and the battle against socialism. It
was also motivated by an equally strong opposition to individual-
ism and liberalism" (1990: 40). McLaughlin states:

> It is argued that despite the dramatic increase in state welfare
> expenditure Catholic social teaching still has a considerable
> role to play in ideologically shaping the contours of social pol-
> icy in Ireland . . . we are also provided with one of the clearest
> examples of how Catholic Corporatism severely restricts
> women's economic, social and reproductive rights (1993: 205).

Thus there is evidence of an obvious corporatist ideology in the form of the Commission on Vocational Organisations (1938) and the formation of the Senate (1937), echoing *Quadragesimo Anno*, "the aim of social policy must therefore be the re-establishment of vocationalist groups" (1931, para 82). Breen et al. (1990) acknowledge the patriarchal and corporatist tendencies in Irish society in the immediate period following the publication of *Quadragesimo Anno*.

THE FORTIES AND FIFTIES

Until 1972, when it was removed after a national referendum, the Roman Catholic Church was guaranteed a special role in the Irish Constitution. A Catholic vision was very much the vision propounded by Eamonn De Valera in the 1940s and his vision encompassed a very particular role for women, which most definitely incorporated their potentiality as mothers:

> That Ireland which we dreamed of would be the home of a people who valued material wealth, only as a basis of right living, of a people who were satisfied with frugal comfort and devoted their leisure to the things of the spirit; a land whose countryside would be bright with cosy homesteads, whose fields and villages would be joyous with the sound of industry, the romping of sturdy children, the contests of athletic youths, the laughter of comely maidens; whose firesides would be the forums of the wisdom of serene old age. It would, in a word, be the home of a people living the life that God desired that men should live (Radio Éireann Broadcast, 17 March 1943).

However, far from this dream coming true, the post-war years in Ireland meant increased prices, more unemployment and emigration. Maguire (1986: 246) refers to the period between 1945 and the early 1950s as a period when there was a heightened interest in Ireland in social policy, noting that pressure for reform had been growing as a result of dissatisfaction with services as they existed together with an interest in the proposed National Health Service in Britain.

The Impact of the Beveridge Report on Ireland

Whyte refers to:

> The wave of discussion that followed the publication in Britain
> of the Beveridge Report . . . by laying down a programme
> through which poverty could be abolished in an entire nation,
> attracted attention far beyond its country of origin (1980: 126).

Pointing to its adaptation in many countries in continental
Europe, Whyte argues that its impact was even stronger in Ireland:

> There was mobility of labour between Ireland and Britain. If
> the standard of British social services rose still further beyond
> those in Ireland, emigration was likely to reach even greater
> heights. Again, such migrants as did return to Ireland were
> likely to become centres of discontent if nothing was done to
> narrow the gap (1980: 126).

Kaim-Caudle reiterates this: ". . . the major changes in social insurance legislation, especially in the years between 1947 and 1953
were much in line with developments in the United Kingdom"
(1967: 39). Even though welfare provision did eventually arrive in
Ireland it came in slowly in an incrementalist way; it never developed to the same extent in Ireland as it did in Britain and remained much less universal.

The old Department of Local Government and Public Health
was replaced by two new departments in 1947: the Department of
Social Welfare, responsible for the provision of income maintenance services, with the Department of Health retaining a minor
role in social welfare provision. In Ireland, a two-tiered income
maintenance system persisted with some of the payments, such as
maternity benefit, based on the insurance/contributory principle.
For those who did not fit into this category, there were means-
tested "assistance payments", such as the maternity grant. Thus,
there was a status-differentiated or a two-tier system, with a no-
tion of the deserving poor versus the needy embedded in the income maintenance system (Carney, 1991; Mills, 1991; Curry,

1993). Differential status is maintained to this day through a system of compulsory social insurance contributions by which eligibility for benefit payments is determined. It is a compulsory insurance against poverty. Alternatively, the assistance scheme calculates payments according to need. It is a residual payment. Status-differentiated payments are gender-biased as they favour the worker who has continuous and full-time employment and in the Ireland of the 1940s and 1950s this always tended to be men. Historically, most women in Ireland, as in many other countries have typically gained welfare entitlements by virtue of their dependency status within the family as wives and mothers. This was based on the assumption that the division of labour followed "naturally" from women's capacity for physiological motherhood. The majority of married women have thus tended to make contributions and draw benefits via their husbands' insurance in accordance with assumptions regarding the existence of a male breadwinner model (Lewis, 1993: 61). Colwill, referring to the "remarkably enduring influence" of the Beveridge Report, points to "its spectacularly successful construction of an ideology of womanhood in particular" (1994: 53).

Writing on welfare regimes, Taylor-Gooby concludes, "conservative/corporatist forces in central government developed a system of occupationally segregated social insurance welfare to insure both middle and working class loyalty and the integration of the trade union movement into the State" (1991: 96). Men who were integrated into the state were guaranteed higher status and influence through citizenship rights while women paid the price. Esping-Andersen's words ring loudly when he refers to the British welfare state: "With its institutionalisation, it becomes a powerful social mechanism which decisively shapes the future" (1990: 221).

A social security system based on the male breadwinner model was essentially discriminatory against women as women were marginalised in the paid labour market and their labour in the home was generally unseen or undervalued. The importance of a contributory record in such a system discriminated against women, who due to their prescribed role as carers in the home were generally unable to develop a contributions record and were thus denied access to benefits.

Colwill highlights Beveridge's demarcation of different types of contributors, for example, self-employed as against employed. This concept of differential status had particular significance for women and with reference to married women's distinct status:

> Patriarchal relations within a capitalist society could thus be faithfully reproduced within the social security system; upon marriage women were quite literally to undergo an economic and social transformation in which the world of work gave way to the world of dependent motherhood (1994: 56).

Income maintenance in Ireland consisted of a social insurance/assistance model with a home assistance safety net, the descendant of outdoor relief. The male breadwinner model assumed that man was the earner and woman the unpaid dependent carer in the home. Single women were discriminated against too: they paid equal contributions to men and they received lower payments. Rates of contribution varied according to age and gender and married women were classed as dependent on their husbands. While married women who remained in the workforce paid lower rates of contribution they received lower payments, reflecting the male breadwinner model:

> Married women living with their husbands need not be included since where the unit is the family, it is the husband's and not the wife's health which it is important to insure. So long as the husband is in good health and able to work adequate provision will be made for the needs of the family, irrespective of the wife's health, whereas when the husband's health fails there is no one to earn wages (Govt. actuaries quoted in Fraser, 1984: 167).

And Taylor-Gooby writes:

> Catholic corporatism regimes tend to define care as largely the province of women and locate it in the informal sector, outside the realm of welfare citizenship . . . (1991: 79).

For the male breadwinner model to succeed, there is a need for women to remain marginal to the paid labour market. Means-tested benefits, lack of childcare provision and community care policies are all based on the principle of subsidiarity and echo Catholic social teaching, i.e. the family is a natural unit and is the basic unit of organisation in society. The family must provide for itself with the state intervening only as a last resort. Subsidiarity has very particular consequences for women. It emphasises the role of mother within the family as the primary caregiver. These sentiments, institutionalised in the 1937 Irish Constitution, echo the 1931 papal encyclical: "it is an injustice and at the same time a grave evil and disturbance of right order to assign to a greater and higher association what lesser and subordinate organisations can do" (1931: para 42).

The Beveridge Report was influential as regards income maintenance but the adoption of a fully comprehensive national health service was never a reality in Ireland. The strength of Catholic social teaching and adherence to the principal of subsidiarity ensured this, as did the vested interests of the medical profession, as evident by the debacle surrounding the Mother and Child Scheme. But before looking at these issues in detail, let us turn to the introduction of Children's Allowances in Ireland, which Lee refers to as "one of the few battles that the forces of resistance lost" (1989: 227). The Beveridge report had advocated a scheme of children's allowances paid out of taxation. The introduction of such allowances, and thus interference in the family, would appear to militate against the principle of subsidiarity (Kennedy, 1994). Bradshaw and Ditch describe the events surrounding the introduction of Children's Allowances in Ireland as "fascinating" (1994: 2). They recount the cases put forward by State and Church in favour and against the introduction of such allowances.

The Introduction of Children's Allowances

In 1926, children's allowances were introduced for civil servants, which Bradshaw and Ditch refer to as "a good example of occupational welfare for securely employed workers" (1994: 2). Farley

(1964) indicates that by the end of 1943 there were Children's Allowance schemes in at least 15 countries, the majority of which were financed by employers and workers. The issue of children's allowances was first raised in 1939 by a member of the Fine Gael party, then in opposition. However, it was not until 1944 that the payment was introduced under the Children's Allowances Act. At first, payments were made in respect of the third and subsequent qualified children, to the head of household. The head of household was generally the father but he could nominate the mother to receive payment. A qualified child was under 16 years, ordinarily resident in the State, not detained in a reformatory or industrial school and not permanently resident in an institution where the cost of their maintenance was defrayed wholly by the governing body, the State or a local authority. Whyte (1980: 103) quotes Dr Dignan, Bishop of Ardfert, who claimed that by both natural and divine law the father was the head of the family and as such bound to maintain the home by himself and that not even the State could relieve him of such duty and privilege. Bradshaw and Ditch (1994: 3) refer to Sean Lemass, who presented the Bill for second reading, arguing for the introduction of such allowances in an effort to meet the needs of large families, as wages are not related to family size but to the issues of productivity, supply and demand in the labour market. While Children's Allowances were introduced without too much church interference, the same could not be said for the Mother and Child Scheme.

Subsidiarity

The Mother and Child Scheme, synonymous with Dr Noel Browne, was undoubtedly a major political crisis and a watershed in social policy as it relates to pregnant women, mothers and their young children. Other writers have documented at length the minutiae of the Scheme and the chronology of events it initiated (Lyons, 1971; Whyte, 1980; Browne, 1986; Barrington, 1987; Lee, 1989).

The Mother and Child Scheme, proposed by the 1947 Health Act, aimed to provide free ante-natal and post-natal care for

mothers, free health care for children up to the age of 16, regardless of means, compulsory school medical inspection, and measures to combat infectious diseases. Tremendous pressure
exercised by both the hierarchy and the medical profession suc-
ceeded in the scheme being modified and eventually adopted under a different administration. Burke, writing in 1993, states:

> By 1950 the medical profession and the Roman Catholic hier-
> archy were totally opposed to the establishment of a free,
> state-run, medical service for mothers and children. To many
> members of the medical profession, the mother and child
> scheme looked like the beginning of a National Health Service
> that would limit their income and autonomy. . . . The govern-
> ment found itself in an impossible position, fighting both the
> Church and the medical profession (1993: 226).

The principal objections of the Catholic hierarchy to the scheme
were that it went against the principle of subsidiarity and under-
mined the privacy of the family:

> . . . the right to provide for the health of children belongs to
> parents not to the state. The State has the right to intervene
> only in a subsidiary capacity, to supplement, not to supplant
> (letter written by James Staunton, Bishop of Ferns, published
> in Browne, 1986, pp. 158–159).

A second reason was the desire to combat the perceived threat of
socialism. It would appear that the hierarchy further objected to
the scheme for fear that contraception may be introduced:

> Education in regard to motherhood includes instruction in re-
> gard to sex relations, chastity and marriage. The State has no
> competence to give instruction in such matters. We regard with
> the greatest apprehension the proposal to give to local medical
> officers the right to tell Catholic girls and women how they
> should behave in regard to this sphere of conduct at once so
> delicate and sacred. Gynaecological care may be and in some
> countries is, interpreted to include provision for birth limitation
> and abortion. We have no guarantee that state officials will re-
> spect Catholic principles in regard to those matters. Doctors

trained in institutions in which we have no confidence may be appointed as medical officers under the proposed services, and may give gynaecological care not in accordance with Catholic principles (letter written by James Staunton, Bishop of Ferns, published in Browne, 1986, pp. 158–159).

Thus, the objections of the Catholic hierarchy and the medical profession to the Mother and Child Scheme were a clear attempt to control women's fertility and call to mind Oakley's sentiments:

> The social control function of the medical and allied professions vis-à-vis women is not a unique case of sexual chauvinism; other social institutions from the law to the national security systems, from the Church to education, from the media to politics also present an image of women which compresses the breadth and variety of their psychologies, lifestyles, satisfactions and dissatisfactions into the basic model of a childish, married, domesticated and neurotic dependent (1981b: 101).

While the Church had its own reasons for blocking the Mother and Child Scheme, it would appear to have used an ally in the guise of the medical profession who feared losing out financially if the Scheme were introduced. To quote once more from the letter of the Bishop of Ferns, "the elimination of private medical practitioners by a state-paid service has not been shown to be necessary or even advantageous to the patient, the public in general or the medical profession" (Browne, 1986: 158–159).

The distinguished Jewish gynaecologist, Michael Solomons concludes that the Church and State colluded with the medical profession in controlling women's fertility through not allowing contraception:

> While the means existed to control fertility, the Irish state lacked the will to allow it. . . . When it came to the prevention of conception and unwanted pregnancy the Church and the state had the Irish people in a moral and legal stranglehold. . . . Meanwhile, the health of women coping with successive pregnancies frequently suffered. When these women looked to the medical

establishment for help, it was not there (Solomons, 1992: 21–22).

The medical profession exercised its strength with its successful intervention as regards the Mother and Child Scheme. Ruth Barrington outlines in detail the fears of the medical profession of losing out financially and their tactical destruction of the Act. Barrington refers to objections that:

> The Bill was a major threat to the private practice of general practitioners who . . . normally made between 70 and 80 per cent of their income from looking after young children. A free service would have dire financial consequences for private doctors and an increase in the number of salaried medical officers would reduce the size of dispensary districts and the scope for private practice (1987: 183).

The foundation of the present Irish maternity services was controversial and steeped in a historical debacle associated with Noel Browne. What developed after Browne's resignation and the fall of the inter-party government, the new Fianna Fáil government's readiness to compromise with the bishops and medical profession, was the Maternity and Infant Care Scheme outlined in the 1953 Health Act and subsequently amended by the 1970 Health Act. Prior to 1953, dispensary medical officers and midwives provided healthcare to poor patients. In some cases, health authorities and voluntary agencies provided clinics and nursing services. It is worth noting that the Mother and Child Scheme, which would have provided free medical care for all pregnant women and mothers and their children, was vetoed at a time when many Irish mothers were under-nourished and suffering from poor health; for example, 75 per cent of mothers giving birth in the Coombe in 1950 were anaemic (Feeney, 1950). To say the least, Irish mothers were not in a favourable position.

The 1953 Act legislated for the provision of a full maternity service (for all women regardless of income) with choice of doctor and midwife and, on payment of an additional fee, choice of hospital or maternity home was assured.

Section 16:

(1) A health authority shall, in accordance with regulations, make available, without charge, medical, surgical, midwifery, hospital and specialist services for attendance to the health of women (being women specified in subsection (2) of this section) in respect of motherhood.

(2) the women referred to in subsection (1) of this section are:

(a) women who are in, or who are dependants of persons in, any of the classes mentioned in subsection (2) of section 15 of this Act,

(b) women by or on behalf of whom such contributions as may be required by regulations have been made towards the cost of the services under this section.

The implementation of this Act was to accelerate the increasing hospitalisation of childbirth and the decline in domiciliary births which can be traced back to 1937, ironically the same year that the Constitution prescribed that woman's place was in the home. Looking at national statistics for domiciliary births as a percentage of national births indicates there has been a sharp decline in the number of women giving birth at home since the 1950s. This is discussed more fully in subsequent chapters.

This period was a particularly painful period for Irish mothers, a period when, as O'Dowd indicates, "the Marian cult contributed to the Catholic idealisation of motherhood while distinguishing the role of procreator and family provider from sex and sexuality" (1987: 13). There were very definitely two distinct groups: those mothers who were married and those mothers who were unmarried. There has emerged in recent years a frightening catalogue of the taboos surrounding extra-marital pregnancy and the associated punishments even though there were changes in both attitudes and services during those decades. Milotte estimated that between 1920 and the mid-1970s more than 100,000 children were born outside of wedlock (1997: 17). He indicates that these "fallen women" had out of necessity to go to the UK, were "married off" or turned to nuns for help, as they were the only people prepared to offer any type of refuge to these women shunned by the remainder of society (1997: 21). Yet, as Milotte indicates, these nuns:

> . . . were part and parcel of the established church, the sole arbitrator of society's moral values. As such, the nuns themselves helped enforce and perpetuate the ethical code that rejected unmarried mothers and banished their hapless offspring. It was a vicious circle (1997: 21).

It is important to acknowledge that such homes had the full approval of Irish society, including the families of the mothers involved and the local authorities which funded them. Milotte describes how young pregnant women approached such homes with great trepidation as such homes had terrible reputations as places of confinement, retribution and punishment. He claims:

> . . . they were not places where the bringing forth of new life was celebrated. The nuns provided secrecy but they exacted a price. Girls and young women entering these institutions, unless they had independent means, had to "work their passage" (1997: 21).

In such institutions, women were labelled, humiliated, made to wear uniforms, have their heads shaved and to carry out the most difficult of physical labour (Finnegan, 2001). Such work often included laundry work, cleaning and scrubbing of convent and church floors. There are reports of one such home in Cork where women who were heavily pregnant worked the convent farm until near the time of delivery. What "leisure time" these women had was often spent praying and making rosary beads, which were sold by the nuns. Media coverage of the Magdalene homes (run independently of the local authorities as voluntary "asylums" and used by all the agencies of the state as penal institutions) and other homes (*Sex in a Cold Climate,* Channel 4, 16 March 1998) disclosed a picture of single mothers, sometimes the victims of sexual abuse themselves, being institutionalised for indefinite periods, which for numerous women meant life. The Magdalene Memorial Group has highlighted how the many women who died in these homes, having spent long lives working there, were buried in unmarked graves, so that even in death they were not vindicated.

Creegan, writing in 1967, refers to the Regina Coeli Hostel in Dublin, run by the Legion of Mary, which she describes as "important as it constitutes the only housing provision available for the unmarried mother who wishes to keep her child" (page 9). For many women, the only hope of freedom was in the form of a marriage proposal. McCarthy (1997) highlights the incarceration of many unmarried pregnant women in lunatic asylums, again committed there by close relatives. Looking at the broader issues around sexuality, she illustrates that women were often sent to such places when they complained of sexual abuse, one such woman being diagnosed as suffering from delusions as she believed that her husband's brothers were abusing both herself and her young daughter. The solution was to incarcerate the mother and leave the daughter to her fate.

Milotte, writing in 1997, exposed the fate of the infants of many of the women incarcerated in these mother and baby homes who as "illegitimate" children were tainted by their status. Referring to Ireland as "a happy hunting ground" for childless couples from the United States, Milotte recalls the events surrounding thousands of foreign adoptions, which, he stresses, continued for 20 years after adoption was introduced in Ireland in 1953 (1997: 15). Referring to the fact that the children sent abroad were referred to as "orphans", this for the majority was, in fact, untrue. He demonstrates that of 330 foreign adoptions in 1952, only three were orphans, the remaining 327 being "illegitimate". Milotte reports that many of the adoptions were organised by nuns, regulated by the Catholic Archbishop of Dublin, John Charles McQuaid, and were facilitated by the State, with the Department of Foreign Affairs issuing passports once the baby was one year old. Milotte says that it is difficult to quantify the number of such adoptions due to the secrecy surrounding the issuing of passports but he estimates that between 1949 and 1973 (the year in which unmarried mothers' allowance was introduced in Ireland) 2,100 children were sent to America. There are no figures available prior to 1949.

EXPANSION

In 1958, the state became involved in economic planning and in the following 14 years three different programmes for economic expansion were implemented. McLaughlin writes that "economic neo-corporatist tendencies emerged in Ireland as elsewhere in western Europe in the post-war period" (1993: 213). Coulter indicates:

> Change has mainly been brought about in the modern Irish state . . . by Government response to pressure. That pressure comes from lobby groups, of which the most successful are the farmers associations, businessmen's organisations, and trade unions and the Catholic Church. Those representing marginalised groups and women have been particularly marginalised in this society and have so far been less successful (1993: 57).

To quote Hernes, "of all of the channels of access to political decision making centres the Corporatist one is the least 'participative', the most hierarchical and the most oligarchical" (1987a: 76). Party politics has never been class-based in Ireland, with nationalist policies dominating class interests. To quote Breen et al.:

> Hence there was a continuous growth of clientelism and coalition building by politicians in an effort to stay in power and to satisfy citizens across the urban/rural divide but at the same time to satisfy the Church which was eager to organise harmonious relations between the social classes to combat the perceived threat of organised labour and socialism (1990: 6).

Esping-Anderson (1990) identifies some of the reasons for corporatism taking hold in a society. These include:

- Late industrialisation, in which guild structures existed until very late, providing a fraternal-type model which already existed

- As a result, status differentiation, hierarchy and privilege were particularly strong, and

- The Catholic Church was directly involved in service provision.

Ireland undoubtedly meets all of these criteria. On the subject of the role of the Catholic Church, Breen et al. state:

> After 1958 the emphasis was on facilitating the implementation of economic planning through the use of consultative bodies and institutionalised negotiation between the "social partners", trade unions, employers and the State, with farmers interests also generally represented. The Catholic Church has not been a participant (Breen, 1990: 6).

Perhaps the Church has not been a formal participant but in a country where the majority are educated in Catholic schools and where the majority of the population is still predominantly Roman Catholic, and where the Catholic Church is involved in service provision, it is safe to assume that the Church is represented in a less formal way. As Cohan states:

> As the chief educator of society the Church has participated in the creation of values that are widely held . . . the Church need not intrude in the political structure because the politicians who are largely responsible for defending such issues happen to hold the same values (1972: 14).

Esping-Andersen associates conservative/corporatist-type societies with a strong Church influence. This would apply to Ireland. As the 1960s came to a close there was evidence of social change in Ireland. Of particular relevance to Irish women of childbearing ages was the introduction in 1963 of the pill as a "cycle regulator" by pharmaceutical companies. The same year saw the publication of *Life Cycle* by Dr Michael Solomons, the first sex education book to be published in Ireland containing anatomically correct diagrams dealing with such subjects as marriage, intercourse, conception, birth, labour, infertility and puberty. It contained no references to contraception or abortion. Six years later in 1969, the Fertility Guidance Company was established in Dublin.

CONCLUSION

This chapter introduced some of the realities of life for mothers in Ireland in the half century following independence. Looking at Ireland as a conservative/corporatist society is beneficial, as it highlights the patriarchal institutional and organisational aspects of state welfare. In the context of a new state struggling to come to terms with a turbulent and persecuted past, extreme poverty and deprivation, it struggled to take control of the future. This included control of women who were designated a very particular role as wife and mother dependent on a male breadwinner, with few rights but many demands, burdens and responsibilities.

What emerges is a bleak and uncompromising picture of life in a patriarchal society, the leading patriarchs being members of the Church, State and the medical profession. Women as mothers were given the tasks of labouring in childbirth, in the home and in the low-paid sectors of the labour market. Women, suffering from ill health, malnutrition and anaemia were expected to bear children frequently and then to rear them in often squalid conditions, providing they were married. Women bearing children outside of wedlock were punished by having little choice other than placing their children for adoption while they themselves were punished by committal to mother and baby homes. Unmarried mothers were criminalised and stigmatised, being referred to as "offenders" or "fallen", and in a society where there was no state payment to enable them support and care for their infants, they had marginal access to the labour market with emigration often being the only option. Women were denied access to abortion and contraception while at the same time chastised and seriously punished for childbearing. Those who bore children both inside and outside wedlock had to be cleansed by the Church by participating in a religious ceremony which again involved humiliation before man and God.

Milotte refers to the decade after the Second World War as "probably the most desolate and gloomy period in modern Irish history" (1997: 17) and he writes:

> Church and state were at one in their determination to enforce a deeply traditional moral code and in the process they displayed what many would see today as an unhealthy obsession with matters sexual, seeking to extend their authority into the bedrooms of the nation. Artificial birth control was outlawed and chastity was demanded of everyone who wasn't married (Milotte, 1997: 17).

Thus, Ireland in 1970 was experiencing the effects of long decades of State and Church working together to reinforce a gendered ideology that believed a woman's place was in the home and her primary role was that of wife and mother, dependent on a male breadwinner. Social policies not only reflected Catholic social teaching but also were shaped by other dominant groups such as the Government, the civil service, the medical and legal professions and the trade unions, all patriarchal groups in nature. However, from the 1970s onwards, there emerged some very powerful social movements such as the women's liberation movement and organisations such as AIM, Cherish, the Irish Family Planning Association, which have acted as powerful catalysts in launching Irish social policies into a new era. Ireland's membership of the European Union has been of paramount importance in the area of social policy and it is in this context, in a climate of change and development, that policies from the 1970s onwards began to develop in a more gender-conscious fashion. It is these policies and influences that the remainder of this book will now proceed to examine.

Chapter Four

CHILDBIRTH IN IRELAND, 1970–2000

Since 1970, Ireland has experienced rapid social change. This period coincided with Ireland becoming a full member of the EU, the second wave of feminism and a reversal of emigration trends. This period was also marked by changes in social policies, which have particular relevance for women during their reproductive years. Motherhood is as much a public issue now as it was in the 1950s when the controversial Mother and Child Scheme was debated. The tremendous energy that has been spent on the issue of reproductive rights since the early 1970s has focused on access to contraception and abortion, to the neglect of the rights of the 50,000 women who give birth in Ireland each year. This chapter focuses on the situation for women who proceed with pregnancy and childbirth. It presents important statistical data for Ireland from 1970 to 2000 in relation to fertility patterns, childbirth and maternity. It highlights trends in service provision and developments in health policy. Before ascertaining who are the women who actually give birth in Ireland, it is useful to outline what services a woman is entitled to during pregnancy and maternity under the Irish health care system.

THE MATERNITY AND INFANT CARE SCHEME

The foundation of the present Irish maternity services was controversial and steeped in the historical debacle associated with Noel Browne TD and the inter-party government of 1948–51, discussed in Chapter Three. The Mother and Child controversy was followed by a period of negotiation and compromise, which produced the Maternity and Infant Care Scheme under the 1953 Health Act. This was superseded by the 1970 Health Act. Eligibility for maternity services was means-tested up until 1991, when under the Health (Amendment) Act eligibility was extended to include all women (this was in line with the extension of eligibility in relation to all hospital services). Currently, the Mother and Infant Care Scheme provides for limited, free, pregnancy-related, general practitioner care for the mother during pregnancy and for six weeks after childbirth, while free care is also provided for the infant for the first six weeks. The Health Strategy (2001) contains an action that this will be increased, when the budgetary climate allows, to six post-natal visits for the infant in the first year of life.

Based on the principle of choice of doctor, the Scheme allows for:

- A first examination for the pregnant woman as near to week 16 as possible but not later than week 28

- Not less than five other examinations before confinement (where possible at least one should be within the last three months)

- Such other examinations and care as deemed necessary by the general practitioner

- The attendance of the doctor on at least one other occasion in the week following the birth

- Such other examinations and after-confinement care as deemed necessary by general practitioner within six weeks

- An examination of the mother at the end of the six weeks

- The supply of articles necessary if the confinement is to take place at home — e.g. lint, cotton, gauze

- The taking of specimens required for investigation

- Medical and surgical services which the general practitioner can provide to the baby during the first six weeks.

Under this scheme, the general practitioner has the right to refuse to accept any patient and it is important to stress that free health care is confined solely to pregnancy-related ailments. The *1997 Report of the Maternity and Infant Care Scheme Review Group* states that "illnesses which occur coincidental but not related to pregnancy should not be provided as part of the scheme free of charge" (Department of Health, 1997b: 15).

In the half-century following the introduction of the Mother and Infant Care Scheme, two reviews were completed. The first review was in 1980 and the findings were reported in the 1981 Department of Health report, *Health Care for Mothers and Infants.* The 1980 survey of all mothers who gave birth from 24–30 November 1980 involved interviews with mothers by public health nurses. The survey covered 93 per cent of births in that week. The report concluded that analysis of statistics showed there was no relation between the take-up of the scheme and decrease in perinatal mortality.

A second review of the Maternity and Infant Care Scheme was undertaken in 1992. It was established to review the current services and its members were expected to complete a review in the context of maternity services generally and make recommendations in a fairly short time, within 12 months (Department of Health, 1997b: 4). The Review Group first met in February 1993. The final report, which was completed in 1994, was not made available to the public until 1997. Initially, the Department of Health claimed the report had not been completed. However, after many approaches by individuals and organisations, including the Home Birth Association and the Irish Association for the Improvement of Maternity Services (IAIMS), the Department of Health admitted that the report had been completed. The Department of Health refused to release the report for public appraisal, arguing that its findings had been included in other Department of Health reports (personal communication, 1996), citing the discussion document *Developing a Policy on Women's Health* (1995). Examination of that report showed no evidence of such inclusion.

Looking at statistics presented in Table 4.1, there is a substantial difference in the numbers of women who actually attend for ante-natal care and post-natal care under the Maternity and Infant Care Scheme and the total number of births recorded. Over 30 per cent of births occur to women not using the scheme for ante-natal care. Prior to 1991 this can be explained in part due to the limited eligibility criteria for that scheme. However, there is still a large difference between the numbers giving birth and those using the scheme. This can best be explained by the fact that a certain number of women do not avail of the scheme. Instead they pay for maternity services on a private basis or avail of VHI or BUPA private medical insurance. The remainder attend maternity units for all ante-natal and post-natal care or avail of the services of a domiciliary midwife.

The 1997 *Report of the Maternity and Infant Care Scheme Review Group* indicates that there is a lack of awareness on the part of both mothers and general practitioners of the existence of the scheme and that among the reasons given by general practitioners (obtained from a limited survey) for not utilising the scheme are inadequate remuneration, too much paper work, difficulty with shared ante-natal care, hospital satellite clinics and lack of knowledge by non-consultant hospital doctors about the scheme. In the course of this research, I encountered one general practitioner who had been practising in excess of 20 years who admitted that she was unaware of the scheme. As women have to complete a form with their GP to avail of services under the scheme, it is possible that a number of women have not done so and hence are not applying for their legal entitlements. It is important to stress that general practitioners have the right to refuse to care for any one individual under this scheme. Some women who expressed a desire to organise a domiciliary birth who have approached their general practitioners to provide ante-natal and post-natal care under the scheme have been refused (as reported at the Home Birth Association Annual Conference, Dublin, 1998).

Table 4.1: Number of Women Attending for Ante-natal Care and Post-natal Care under the Maternity and Infant Care Scheme in Ireland for Selected Years, 1978-1997 (latest available data)

Year	Total Number of Live Births (1)	Number Receiving Ante-natal Care (2)	Ante-natal Care (2) as a % of All Births (1) (3)	Number Receiving Post-natal Care (4)	Post-natal Care Attendance as % of All Those Attending Ante-natal Care (5)
1978	70,299	30,299	43.1	26,158	86.3
1979	72,539	29,199	40.2	25,207	86.3
1980	74,064	32,897	44.4	28,661	87.1
1981	72,158	30,858	42.8	26,610	86.2
1982	70,843	30,840	43.5	28,298	91.7
1984	64,062	27,266	42.6	24,793	90.9
1985	62,388	26,538	42.5	23,267	87.7
1986	61,620	26,750	43.4	23,890	89
1987	58,433	25,723	44.0	23,082	90
1988	54,600	23,895	43.8	21,662	91
1989	52,018	23,912	46.0	21,286	89
1990	53,044	24,150	45.5	21,422	89
1991*	52,718	n/a	n/a	n/a	n/a

Table 4.1 cont'd

Year	Total Number of Live Births (1)	Number Receiving Ante-natal Care (2)	Ante-natal Care (2) as a % of All Births (1) (3)	Number Receiving Post-natal Care (4)	Post-natal Care Attendance as % of All Those Attending Ante-natal Care (5)
1992	51,089	27,809	54.4	25,134	90
1993	49,461	26,683	53.9	24,021	90
1994	47,928	28,512	59.5	25,619	90
1995	48,530	29,922	61.7	26,291	88
1996	50,655	33,214	65.6	30,073	91
1997	52,775	35,311	66.9	33,165	94

*From 1991 eligibility for the Maternity and Infant Care Scheme was extended to all women under the 1991 Health (Amendment) Act.

n/a denotes not available

Source: Compiled by author from *Vital Statistics* (Central Statistics Office) and *Health Statistics* (Department of Health) for selected years 1978-1997 from latest available data at time of going to print.

Table 4.1 presents data on the number of women attending for ante-natal care and post-natal care under the Maternity and Infant Care Scheme. Attendance means appearing once during pregnancy or during the six weeks after childbirth. This is a very limited definition of "care". The numbers of those attending for ante-natal care as a proportion of all births has increased notably since 1991, the year in which eligibility was extended to cover all mothers. A possible explanation for the fact that fewer women attend for post-natal care than ante-natal care may be that women are more concerned for their own health when they are pregnant, as they feel that their own health status will affect that of the baby. Another possible explanation is the perceived inadequacy of post-natal care and the difficulty of women in accessing health services when they are coming to terms with the complexities of the first weeks of motherhood. This important topic is addressed in Chapter Seven.

DATA ON MOTHERS

The majority of babies, over 90 per cent, are born to women in the 15–49 year age group. In Ireland in 2000 there were 993,800 women in this age group, an increase of 366,800 since 1971 (Table 4.2). Thus the number of potential users of Irish maternity services has increased considerably in this period.

Table 4.2: Number of Women Aged 15-49 for Selected Years in Ireland, 1971-2000

Year	Number of Women
1971	627,000
1981	780,000
1986	839,000
1991	869,000
1996	934,170
2000	993,800*

Source: Compiled by author from Census of Population for 1971, 1981, 1986, 1991, 1996 (figure for 2000 is provisional and was provided by the CSO).

Age-specific fertility rates for the 1970–2000 period indicates a reduction for all age cohorts except for the 15–19 age group which shows an increase of 3.1 per 1,000 for the 30–year period 1970–2000 (Table 4.3). The fertility rate for this age cohort is important and will be addressed later on in the context of risk for young mothers during childbirth. At the other end of the scale, the age-specific fertility rate for mothers aged 35 to 49, also classified as a high-risk group, has decreased from 180.9 in 1970 to 86.6 in 2000. The total period fertility rate for this period has also shown a decline from 3.87 in 1970 to 1.89 in 2000 (see Glossary for definitions).

Table 4.3: Age-specific Fertility Rate and Total Period Fertility Rate (TPFR) for Women in Ireland for Selected Years 1970–2000

Year	Live Births per 1,000 Females at Specified Ages							
	15–19	*20–24*	*25–29*	*30–34*	*35–39*	*40–44*	*45–49*	*TPFR*
1970	16.3	145.5	228.7	201.9	131.9	45.3	3.7	3.87
1975	22.8	138.6	216.1	162.2	100.1	36.8	2.6	3.40
1981	22.2	117.4	190.3	161.5	93.6	26.5	2.4	3.07
1986	15.4	83.1	154.3	139.0	73.4	21.2	1.5	2.45
1987	16.1	75.4	147.9	132.3	68.6	19.8	1.3	2.31
1988	15.1	69.6	140.9	125.5	63.1	17.8	1.1	2.17
1989	14.8	64.0	134.5	122.0	62.4	17.0	1.1	2.08
1990	16.7	63.3	137.6	126.2	63.0	15.4	1.1	2.12
1991	17.2	63.6	131.6	124.6	63.6	15.2	1.0	2.08
1992	17.2	58.8	125.8	124.5	61.6	14.6	0.8	2.02
1993	17.2	52.4	116.7	125.2	58.7	14.1	0.9	1.93
1994	15.0	50.7	112.5	119.6	58.6	12.8	0.7	1.85
1995	15.1	50.3	106.7	123.5	60.3	13.11	0.8	1.85
1996	16.7	52.2	105.3	127.1	63.9	11.8	0.6	1.89
1997	17.5	50.6	105.4	132.9	67.2	13.5	0.8	1.94
1998	19.1	51.2	100.7	134.1	70.4	13.5	0.6	1.95
1999	20.0	49.1	95.9	133.4	70.2	13.1	0.6	1.91
2000	19.4	48.7	90.7	132.5	72.5	13.6	0.5	1.89

Source: Central Statistics Office (vital statistics for selected years)

Table 4.4: Number of Live Births to Women at Specified Ages as a Percentage of Total Live Births for Selected Years in Ireland 1971-2000

Year	15 and Under	16	17	18	19	20	21	22	23	24	Total of 24 and Under	As a % of All Births
1970	28	106	324	613	1,038	1,738	2,385	3,111	3,653	3,899	16,895	26.2
1975	60	197	465	972	1,561	2,280	3,637	3,394	3,880	4,097	19,543	29.1
1980	63	196	533	1,023	1,765	2,308	2,708	3,341	3,882	4,258	20,077	27.1
1985	41	155	413	803	1,229	1,619	1,914	2,415	2,917	3,313	14,819	23.8
1990	66	178	458	790	1,176	1,239	1,345	1,588	1,801	2,177	10,818	20.4
1991	55	195	456	894	1,194	1,356	1,402	1,596	1,802	2,042	10,992	20.86
1992	45	189	472	801	1,214	1,360	1,322	1,527	1,754	1,997	10,681	20.7
1993	57	177	450	799	1,153	1,236	1,320	1,378	1,612	1,873	10,056	20.9
1994	67	177	388	738	1,006	1,133	1,276	1,390	1,435	1,791	9,401	19.6
1995	57	209	435	771	1,010	1,155	1,295	1,398	1,525	1,731	9,586	19.8
2000	65	212	511	995	1,351	1,549	1,510	1,562	1,574	1,667	10,996	20.3

Source: Compiled by author from *Vital Statistics* (CSO) for selected years.

Looking at Table 4.4, a startling figure is that the number of young women and girls giving birth aged 16 years and under are victims of "statutory rape". In 2000, the figure was 277 births. The number of births to women and girls aged 24 years and under as a proportion of all births has decreased from 26.2 per cent (16,895) in 1970 to 20.3 per cent (10,996) in 2000. The number of births to young women aged 20 to 24 has decreased. On the other hand, the numbers of births in the lower age groups, 19 years and under, have all increased. And for those aged 16 and under, the numbers have more than doubled. This has implications for maternity services, as there is an acceptance by the medical profession that teenage mothers are at particular risk in childbirth. It also has implications for support services for teenage mothers (Flanagan and Richardson, 1992).

Statistics demonstrate that there is also a change in the age profile of primaparae or first-time mothers (Table 4.5). This group too is judged by obstetric science to be a high-risk group. Statistics on age of mother at first maternity show a 7.1 per cent reduction in mothers aged under 25 years and a smaller decrease of 0.4 per cent in the proportion of mothers aged 35 years and over between 1971 and 1998 (Table 4.6). This indicates that the fertility period has decreased for women, in that women are now more likely to give birth during a shorter span of years than previously (Table 4.5). In 1971, 52.8 per cent of first births were to women aged between 25 and 35, while in 1998 the figure was 59.5 per cent. It has tended to fluctuate around 60 per cent, a trend that has developed since the mid-1980s, and is perhaps an indication of mothers attempting to reconcile childbearing and childcare with participation in the labour market (as is explored later in this book).

In 1971, 28.3 per cent of women who gave birth were first-time mothers. The figure for 2000 was 40.5 per cent. This increase in first-time mothers has implications for support services for women. It is at first childbirth that women have to learn the skills of parentcraft, accomplish the difficult skill of breastfeeding and begin to reconcile employment with childcare responsibilities. In modern society, first-time motherhood has tended to take on major significance as a "rite of passage" for women. Ann Oakley writes:

> First-time motherhood calls for massive changes . . . becoming a mother is more than a change of job; it involves reorganising one's entire personality. For there is a chasm between mothers' needs and children's needs that mothers have to bridge (1979: 12).

Table 4.5: Age at First Maternity in Ireland for Selected Years, 1970–1998

Year	% of First Births to Mothers under 25	% of First Births to Mothers Aged 25–34 Years	% of First Births to Mothers 35 and Over	Total Live Births
1971	27.1	52.8	20.1	67,551
1974	28.8	53.8	17.4	68,907
1976	28.6	55.6	15.8	67,718
1978	27.5	57.1	15.4	70,299
1980	27.4	57.3	15.3	74,064
1981	27.0	57.6	15.4	72,158
1982	26.1	58.0	15.9	70,843
1983	25.8	58.2	16.3	67,117
1984	25.6	58.0	16.4	64,062
1985	17.4	66.0	16.6	62,388
1986	23.5	59.5	17.0	61,620
1988	22.0	61.0	17.0	54,600
1990	20.3	62.5	17.2	53,044
1992	20.7	61.5	17.8	51,089
1993	20.5	61.4	18.1	49,461
1994	19.6	62.2	18.22	47,928
1995	19.75	61.4	18.9	48,530
1998	20.0	59.5	20.5	53,551

Source: Table compiled by author from Department of Health Statistics for selected years 1971–1998.

Table 4.6: Previous Children at Maternity in Ireland for Selected Years, 1970–2000

Year	% of Births to Mothers with No Previous Children (1)	% of Births to Mothers with 1–3 Previous Children (2)	% of Births to Mothers with 4+ Previous Children (3)	Total
1971	28.3	49.9	21.8	67,551
1974	29.9	52.4	17.7	68,907
1978	30.7	52.6	16.7	72,299
1980	29.2	55.8	15.3	74,064
1981	28.6	56.6	14.8	72,158
1982	28.4	56.1	15.5	70,843
1983	28.7	56.5	14.7	67,117
1984	29.7	56.0	14.3	64,062
1985	29.9	56.6	13.5	62,388
1986	30.5	56.3	13.2	61,620
1990	33.3	56.2	10.5	53,044
1992	35.4	55.4	9.2	51,089
1993	35.4	56.4	8.2	49,461
1994	35.2	56.3	7.3	47,928
1995	36.3	56.6	6.7	48,530
1996	37.9	55.7	6.1	50,665
1997	38.3	55.9	5.1	52,775
1998	39.4	55.3	5.0	53,969
1999	40.5	54.4	4.8	53,924
2000	40.5	54.4	4.5	54,239

Source: Compiled from *Vital Statistics* (CSO) for selected years.

In the 32 years since 1970, there has been a dramatic decline in family size in Ireland. The number of women giving birth who already had four or more children decreased from 21.8 per cent in 1971 to 4.5 per cent in 2000, as illustrated in Table 4.6. This has serious implications for maternity services, as parity is viewed as a risk factor by obstetric science. This issue too is explored later in this book.

While the birth rate in Ireland varied little prior to 1971, from then on it fell until the mid-1990s when it began to rise again. It is interesting to note that the contraceptive pill became available as a "cycle regulator" in Ireland in the 1960s (Solomons, 1992) and Mary Robinson began her campaign in the Oireachtas to repeal the laws banning contraception in 1971, a campaign that would not bear fruition until 1985. Table 4.7 shows that in 1971 there were 22.7 births per thousand population. In 1994, the birth rate reached a low of 13.4. In 1981, the birth rate had fallen to 21.0 births per thousand, while the actual number of births rose but by 1994 the total number of live births had fallen to 47,928. However, looking at the birth rate in a European context, Ireland still has one of the highest national birth rates and at 14.3 is above the EU average of 10.6 (Eurostat, 1999). There has been a steady increase in the number of births since 1995, with 54,239 births in 2000. This rise in the number of births has implications for the provision of maternity services. However, there are fewer births than occurred in the early to mid-1980s. Remarkably, in 1981 there were 72,158 births in Ireland, 17,919 more than in 2000. This is important in the light of constant requests from the Dublin maternity hospitals for extra resources because of "unprecedented demands". This figure would challenge such requests.

Table 4.7: Birth Rate: Births per 1,000 of Population in Ireland for Selected Years, 1951–2000

Year	Ireland	Total Live Births
1951	21.2	62,878
1961	21.2	59,825
1971	22.7	67,551
1981	21.0	72,158
1982	20.3	70,843
1983	19.1	67,117
1884	18.2	64,062
1985	17.6	62,388
1986	17.4	61,620
1987	16.5	58,433
1988	15.4	54,600
1989	14.8	52,076
1990	15.1	53,044
1991	15.0	52,718
1992	14.4	51,089
1993	13.9	49,461
1994	13.4	47,928
1995	13.5	48,530
1996	14.0	50,665
1997	14.4	52,775
1998	14.5	53,551
1999	14.2	53,354
2000	14.3	54,239

Source: Central Statistics Office

There has been a major decline in maternal mortality since the 1970s. Maternal mortality patterns show a decline from 25 per 100,000 births in 1970 to 2 per 100,000 births in 2000 (Table 4.8). Factors contributing to this decline include age of mother when giving birth, lower parity, improvements in women's general health and better socio-economic conditions (Tew, 1995).

Table 4.8: Maternal Mortality in Ireland for Selected Years, 1970–2000

Year	Total Numbers of Maternal Deaths	Rate per 100,000 Live and Still-births	Total Live Births
1970	17	25.0	64,382
1971	17	25.0	67,551
1972	27	39.4	68,527
1973	8	11.6	68,713
1978	12	17.6	70,299
1979	10	14	72,539
1980	4	5.4	74,064
1981	3	4.2	72,158
1982	3	4.2	70,843
1983	8	11.9	67,117
1984	3	4.7	64,062
1985	5	8.0	62,388
1986	4	6.5	61,620
1987	1	1.7	58,433
1988	2	3.7	54,600
1990	3	5.7	53,044
1991	2	3.8	52,718
1992	1	1.9	51,089
1993	0	0	49,461
1994	1	2	47,928
1995	–	–	48,530
1996	3	6	50,665
1997	3	6	52,775
1998	2	4	53,551
1999	1	2	53,354
2000	1	2	54,239

Source: Compiled by author from Department of Health statistics for selected years.

Over the period from 1971 to 2000 there has been an increase in both the number and the percentage of births occurring outside marriage from 2.7 per cent of live births in 1971 to 31.8 per cent in 2000 (Table 4.9). This coincides with a period of rapid social change in Ireland, including a change in attitudes towards women who give birth outside marriage (McCarthy, 1995a), specific policy changes such as the Status of Children Act (1987) and the introduction of Unmarried Mothers Allowance in 1973 (Flanagan and Richardson, 1992; Conroy, 1993, 1997), as well as a rise in consensual unions (Flanagan and Richardson, 1992; Conroy, 1997). Some of these issues are addressed in subsequent chapters.

Table 4.9: Non-marital Births in Ireland as a Percentage of Total Live Births, 1971–2000

Year	Total Number of Non-marital Births	% of Non-marital Births	Total Number of Live Births
1971	1,824	2.7	67,551
1972	1,959	2.9	68,527
1973	2,189	3.2	68,713
1974	2,343	3.4	68,907
1975	2,485	3.7	67,178
1976	2,553	3.8	67,718
1977	2,893	4.2	68,892
1978	3,023	4.3	70,299
1979	3,328	4.5	72,539
1980	3,719	4.5	74,064
1981	3,911	5.4	72,158
1982	4,357	6.2	70,843
1983	4,551	6.8	67,117
1984	5,118	8.0	64,062
1985	5,284	8.5	62,388
1986	5,946	9.7	61,620

Year	Total Number of Non-marital Births	% of Non-marital Births	Total Number of Live Births
1987	6,346	10.9	58,433
1988	5,930	10.9	54,600
1989	6,181	11.9	52,018
1990	6,835	12.9	53,044
1991	7,704	14.6	52,718
1992	9,303	18.2	51,089
1993	9,608	19.4	49,461
1994	9,450	19.7	47,928
1995	10,788	22.2	48,530
2000	17,235	31.8	54,239

Source: *Vital Statistics* (Central Statistics Office) for selected years, 1971–2000

Another important issue concerns those women whose pregnancies do not result in childbirth, that is, the women who experience miscarriage and abortion and who are not included in the fertility data on which planning is based (see notes to Table 4.3). It is impossible to estimate the exact number of women whose pregnancies end in miscarriage, as many women who miscarry are not aware that they are doing so. With regard to abortion, Irish women have generally availed of services in Britain due to the fact that abortion in Ireland is unavailable (Smyth, 1993; Conroy, 1997; Mahon et al., 1998). Figures again are inconclusive but statistics for women availing of abortion services in Britain who give Irish addresses are as shown in Table 4.10.

Table 4.10: Number of Terminations for Women Giving Irish Addresses in Britain for Selected Years, 1981-2000

Year	Number of Women
1981	3,603
1982	3,650
1983	3,677
1984	3,946
1985	3,888
1986	3,918
1987	3,673
1988	3,839
1989	3,721
1990	4,064
1991	4,154
1992	4,254
1993	4,402
1994	4,590
1995	4,532
2000	6,381
2001	6,625

Source: Office of Population Census and Statistics (2001) London.

PLACE OF BIRTH

Where a woman gives birth is important from the point of view of the woman herself and her child and in the context of the State and the social policies required. There has been a steady decline in domiciliary births in Ireland in the second half of this century (Table 4.11), reflecting developments in health policy. This decline in domiciliary births has continued since the 1970s. In 1955, the year after the Maternity and Infant Care Scheme was introduced, over a third of births in Ireland were domiciliary. The proportion of all births which were domiciliary in 1999 was less than one per cent and amounted to only 262 births or fewer than six a week (latest available figure).

Table 4.11: Domiciliary Births as a Percentage of All Live Births, Number of Domiciliary and Hospital Births and Total Live Births in Ireland for Selected Years, 1955–2000

Year	Domiciliary %	Domiciliary Births	Hospital Births	Total Live Births
1955	33.5	20,665	40,957	61,622
1957	29.5	18,100	43,142	61,242
1962	17.6	10,864	50,918	61,782
1966	8.5	5,304	56,911	62,215
1967	6.8	4,139	57,168	61,307
1969	4.0	2,517	60,395	62,912
1970	3.0	1,883	62,499	64,382
1971	2.1	1,447	66,104	67,551
1972	1.8	1,150	67,377	68,527
1973	1.2	830	67,883	68,713
1974	0.8	535	68,372	68,907
1978	0.4	259	70,040	70,299
1979	0.4	262	72,277	72,539
1980	0.3	202	73,862	74,064
1981	0.3	210	71,948	72,158
1982	0.3	232	70,611	70,843
1983	0.3	206	66,911	67,117
1984	0.3	182	63,880	64,062
1985	0.3	165	62,223	62,388
1986	0.3	196	61,424	61,620
1987	0.3	165	58,268	58,433
1988	0.3	188	54,412	54,600
1989	0.3	152	51,924	52,018
1990	0.3	147	53,165	53,044
1991	0.3	178	52,445	52,718
1992	0.3	144	50,893	51,089
1993	0.3	140	49,130	49,461
1994	0.4	202	47,727	47,928

Year	Domiciliary %	Domiciliary Births	Hospital Births	Total Live Births
1995	0.4	189	48,341	48,530
1996	0.4	212	50443	50,655
1997	0.5	271	53504	52,775
1998	0.4	222	53329	53,551
1999	0.5	262	53092	53,354

Source: Compiled by author from Department of Health Statistics for selected years, 1955–1999

Since the late 1970s, smaller maternity units have been closed down as a result of a government policy (addressed in Chapter Six) that all births should take place in obstetric-staffed maternity units. This has coincided with an increase in the number of births in larger maternity units (Table 4.12).

Table 4.12: Percentage Distribution of All Births by Size (annual number of births) of Maternity Units 1978, 1983 and 1993

Annual Number of Births Occurring in Hospital Size of Unit (number of births)	1978 % of Total Births	1983 % of Total Births	1993 % of Total Births
4,000 and over	37.7	37	36.9
2,000 to 3,999	21.9	29.9	17.0
1,500 to 1,999	14.2	10.2	16.9
1,000 to 1,499	5.6	11.3	23.7
500 to 999	9.7	7.0	2.7
100 to 499	8.5	1.9	2.2
fewer than 100	1.6	1.0	0.3
Domiciliary	0.8	1.4	0.3

Source: *Health Statistics*, Department of Health, 1978, 1983 and 1993 (latest available data).

Parallel to the increased hospitalisation of childbirth has come an increased medicalisation and a trend towards more obstetric interventions, i.e. the active management of labour as opposed to active labour. Interventions include episiotomies, caesarean sections and epidurals. This trend is further analysed in later chapters, but an indication of the increased medicalisation of childbirth is presented here. In particular, statistics on caesarean sections, epidurals and episiotomies are presented. For this purpose, the clinical reports of the Coombe Women's Hospital, the National Maternity Hospital and the Rotunda were collated and analysed (see Table 4.13). More than 30 per cent of births have taken place in these three hospitals in every year since 1978. In 2000, the figure was 40 per cent.

In both the National Maternity Hospital and the Coombe in 2000 there were more than 20 babies born every 24 hours, whereas in the Rotunda there were 17 births. The proportion of births in these three hospitals has risen from 27.37 per cent of all births in 1970 to 40 per cent in 2000. The number of births in each of these three hospitals is now higher than in 1970. In all three hospitals, there was a sizeable increase in the number of births in the late 1970s, reflecting the higher number of births nationally during that period. However, the number of births in the three units did not have a parallel increase in births as a proportion of all births. In 1981, there were 8,964 births in the National Maternity Hospital, representing 24.6 births every 24 hours or slightly more than one birth per hour. This is interesting in the light of evidence presented in the next chapter on the active management of labour which was gaining strength in that hospital at the time and was seen as a strategy to deal with the "bottle-neck of the labour ward" (O'Driscoll, 1993).

Table 4.13: Annual Numbers of Births (live plus late fetal deaths) for the Coombe, the National Maternity Hospital and the Rotunda for the years 1970-2000 as a Percentage of All Births in the State

Year	Coombe	National Maternity Hospital	Rotunda	Total Births for the Three Hospitals	National (live plus late fetal deaths)	Total for Three Hospitals as a % of National Total
1970	5,681	6,255	5,936	17,872	65,286	27.37
1971	6,726	7,083	4,912	18,721	68,432	27.36
1972	7,856	7,252	4,969	19,804	69,428	28.52
1973	7,631	7,315	5,054	20,000	69,542	28.76
1974	77,21	7,676	5,174	20,571	69,774	29.48
1975	7,301	7,430	5,310	20,041	67,952	29.49
1976	7,111	7,553	5,713	20,387	68,483	29.77
1977	7,099	7,590	6,120	20,819	69,649	29.89
1978	7,516	8,101	6,204	21,821	70,958	30.75
1979	7,642	8,450	6,330	22,422	73,223	30.62
1980	7,685	8,849	6,515	23,049	74,745	30.84
1981	7,265	8,964	6,175	22,404	72,758	30.79
1982	6,884	8,653	6,102	21,639	71,414	30.30
1983	6,435	8,159	5,797	20,391	67,698	30.12
1984	6,280	7,879	5,611	19,770	64,604	30.60

Year	Coombe	National Maternity Hospital	Rotunda	Total Births for the Three Hospitals	National (live plus late fetal deaths)	Total for Three Hospitals as a % of National Total
1985	6,354	7,512	5,709	19,575	62,904	31.12
1986	6,240	7,150	5,910	19,300	62,099	31.08
1987	6,507	6,725	5,631	18,863	58,849	32.05
1988	7,049	7,069	5,804	19,922	54,986	36.23
1989	6,664	6,375	5,893	18,932	52,348	36.16
1990	6,854	6,328	5,923	19,105	53,371	35.63
1991	6,987	6,277	6,129	19,393	53,019	36.58
1992	6,571	6,293	5,692	18,556	51,374	36.12
1993	6,369	6,378	5,563	18,310	49,752	36.80
1994	6,539	6,321	5,576	18,436	48,225	38.23
1995	6,388	6,718	5,595	18,710	48,740	38.39
1996	6,513	7,275	5,857	19,645	50,989	38.52
1997	6,854	7,682	6,223	20,759	53,143	30.06
1998	6,997	7,948	6,387	21,332	53,879	39.59
1999	7,067	7,659	6,334	21,060	53,665	39.24

Source: Compiled by author from annual clinical reports of the Coombe, the National Maternity and the Rotunda Hospitals 1970-1999

In these three hospitals, maternal mortality (defined as the death of a woman while pregnant or within 42 days of termination of pregnancy) is now a rare occurrence (Table 4.14). National figures for maternal mortality have also declined from 17 in 1970 to 1 in 2000 (Table 4.8).

Table 4.14: Maternal Mortality in the Coombe, the National Maternity and the Rotunda Hospitals for Selected Years, 1970–2000

Year	Coombe Hospital	Nat. Maternity Hospital	Rotunda Hospital	National
1970	3	0	n/a	17
1971	1	4	n/a	15
1978	2	3	1	10
1979	2	2	1	10
1980	1	0	2	4
1981	1	3	0	3
1982	1	0	0	3
1983	2	1	3	n/a
1984	1	1	2	3
1985	1	1	0	5
1986	0	0	2	4
1987	2	2	0	1
1990	1	1	0	3
1991	1	2	0	2
1992	1	0	0	1
1993	0	0	1	0
1994	0	0	0	1
1995	1	0	1	–
1996	0	0	0	3
1997	0	1	1	3
1998	2	0	0	2
1999	1	2	2	1
2000	0	0	0	1

Source: Complied by author from annual clinical reports of the Coombe, the National Maternity and the Rotunda Hospitals, 1970–2000 and *Health Statistics*, Department of Health, selected years. n/a denotes not available.

Looking at national statistics for caesarean sections (Table 4.15), which, apart from terminations, is probably the most extreme obstetric intervention, there has been an increase in caesarean sections from 7.41 per cent to 20.6 per cent between 1984 and 1999 (the latest date for which statistics are available).

Table 4.15: Caesarean Sections in Irish Maternity Units, 1984–99

Year	Caesarean Births (%)	Total Births
1984	7.41	64,062
1985	7.78	62,388
1986	8.5	61,620
1987	8.9	58,433
1988	9.6	54,600
1989	10.0	52,018
1990	10.5	53,044
1991	11.8	52,442
1992	12.2	51,089
1999	20.6	53,354

Source: *Perinatal Statistics* (Department of Health) for selected years 1984–1992 (1999 figure supplied by ESRI HIPE Unit).

In the context of the national rate of caesarean sections, the rates in the Coombe, the National Maternity Hospital and the Rotunda (Table 4.16) for 1992 were 12.0 per cent, 8.5 per cent and 13.7 per cent respectively. So, in that year the rate in the Rotunda was above the national average while that in the Coombe was close to the national average and the National Maternity Hospital was slightly below. Looking at statistics for 1999, the Rotunda Hospital had a rate of 25.5 per cent (Table 4.16), considerably more than either the Coombe or the National Maternity Hospital and above the national average (Table 4.15). Furthermore, the Rotunda's caesarean rate more than doubled since 1978 when it was 8.9 per cent. In the Coombe, the caesarean rate increased from 7.3 per cent in 1978 to 16.9 per cent in 2000, and in the National Maternity Hospital the rate again more than trebled from 4.7 per cent in 1978 to 14.2 per cent in 2000. Interestingly, these statistics show a difference in rates of caesareans: 25.5 per cent in the Rotunda, 16.9 per cent in the Coombe and 14.2 per cent in the National Maternity Hospital. This raises questions as to why such a serious intervention as caesarean should have such different rates in the three maternity units in this study (this issue will be addressed in Chapter Six).

Table 4.16: Trends in Caesarean Section Rate as a Proportion of All Live Births for Selected Years between 1970 and 2000

Year	Coombe Hospital (%)	Nat. Maternity Hospital (%)	Rotunda Hospital (%)
1978	7.3	4.7	8.9
1981	8.7	5.5	6.9
1982	8.5	5.2	7.8
1983	7.6	6	8.9
1984	6.3	4.2	11.7
1985	7.8	5.1	11.1
1986	8.5	5.3	11.7
1987	9.6	5.9	12.7
1988	9.9	6.1	12
1989	11.5	6.5	11.8
1990	11.3	8.5	11.7
1991	11.3	9	14.2
1992	12	8.5	13.7
1993	12.9	9.8	15.2
1994	12.6	8.8	16.4
1995	12.6	10.3	18.3
1996	14.5	10.8	19.8
1997	13.8	10.8	21.9
1998	14.7	12.8	24.2
1999	16.3	12.9	25.1
2000	16.9	14.2	25.5

Source: Compiled by author from annual clinical reports for the Coombe, the National Maternity Hospital and the Rotunda 1970–2000

Similar questions need to be raised regarding other obstetric interventions including episiotomies (Table 4.17), and epidurals (Table 4.18), which have also risen considerably.

Table 4.17: Episiotomy Rate: Primagravidae and Multigravidae in the Coombe, the National Maternity and the Rotunda Hospitals, 1998

Episiotomy Rate (%)	Coombe Hospital (%)	Nat. Maternity Hospital (%)	Rotunda Hospital (%)
Primagravidae	41	52	n/a
Multigravidae	10	12	n/a
Total Prima and Multips	n/a	n/a	35

Source: Extracted from *Preparing Together for Birth and Beyond: A Consumer Guide to the Maternity Services in Ireland*, Cuidiú Irish Childbirth Trust (1999).

Table 4.18: Epidural Rates in the Coombe, the National Maternity and the Rotunda Hospitals for Selected Years, 1970–2000

Year	Coombe Hospital (%)	Nat. Maternity Hospital (%)	Rotunda Hospital (%)
1974	n/a	n/a	1.3
1975	n/a	n/a	3
1980	n/a	n/a	17.2
1986	19.3	4.4	37.2
1992	45.4	30.7	54
1993	43	36.4	56
1995	45.1	47.6	66.7
2000	51.4	48.6	52.5

Source: Compiled by author from annual clinical records for the Coombe, the National Maternity Hospital and the Rotunda Hospitals, 1970–2000

Looking at statistics for episiotomies for 1999, first-time mothers in the Coombe (41 per cent) were less likely to be subjected to this intervention than in the National Maternity Hospital, where the procedure was done to more than half of all first time mothers (52 per cent). The figures for the Rotunda are for both primagravidae and multiparous combined, a rate of 35 per cent. However, statistics show multigravidae mothers in the National Maternity Hospital were more likely to be subjected to episiotomies than in the Coombe. These figures should be read in conjunction with the rates for caesarean sections, as those women will not have given birth vaginally.

Statistics on the use of epidurals again show differences for all three hospitals (Table 4.18). Overall, the epidural rate has risen dramatically. Again, the Rotunda comes top of the league table with 52.5 per cent of mothers receiving epidurals in 2000, while the rates for the Coombe and the National Maternity Hospital are 51.4 per cent and 48.6 per cent respectively.

It is interesting to read these figures in the context of the increased hospitalisation of childbirth (Table 4.11) and the decline in domiciliary births. Women giving birth at home do not experience any of the above procedures.

DATA ON INFANTS

Looking at the outcome of birth, i.e. perinatal, neonatal and infant mortality rates, one observes that these have steadily declined since 1971 (Table 4.19) (see glossary for definitions). Despite dramatic improvements in neo-natal care, babies born before 26 weeks gestation still have only a 50 per cent survival rate and neonatal death rates remain high up until 28–30 weeks (Chamberlain, 1995). This is very important as risk of neonatal death is often suggested as a reason why all births should take place in a maternity hospital. Many of the risk factors associated with perinatal mortality relate to social conditions — social class, racial origin and smoking (Chamberlain et al., 1995: 360–361).

Table 4.19: Perinatal, Neonatal and Infant Mortality Rates in Ireland, 1971-2000

Year	Perinatal per 1,000 Live and Stillbirths	Neonatal per 1,000 Live Births	Infant per 1,000 Live Births
1971	22.8	12.2	17.97
1972	23.2	12.1	18.04
1973	22.9	12.7	17.9
1974	22.0	11.6	17.8
1975	21.5	12	17.5
1976	19.7	10.4	15.5
1977	19.2	9.9	15.5
1978	17.6	9.8	14.8
1979	16.2	8.4	12.8
1980	14.8	6.7	11.1
1981	10.6	6.7	10.6
1982	10.5	6.6	10.5
1983	9.8	5.8	9.8
1984	10.1	6.3	13.4
1985	8.9	5.4	13.7
1987	7.4	3.9	12.3
1989	9.2	5.5	11.8
1990	10.4	4.6	8.2
1991	8.2	5.4	11.3
1992	6.6	4.3	10.2
1993	5.9	4.0	9.4
1994	9.4	4.0	5.9
1995	9.1	4.6	6.3
1996	8.6	4.1	6.0
1997	8.1	3.5	6.1
1998	8.1	4.3	5.9
1999	7.5	3.9	5.9

Source: Compiled by author from Department of Health statistics for selected years, 1971–1999 (latest available data).

CONCLUSION

This chapter identifies some statistical trends reflecting childbirth patterns in Ireland since the 1970s. The Maternity and Infant Care Scheme has been in existence since 1954 and has been reviewed twice (Department of Health, 1981, 1997b). Both reviews recommend that all births should take place in obstetric-staffed maternity units and this is reflected in numbers of women giving birth at home, with figures decreasing from 33.5 per cent of all births (20,665 births) in 1955 to 0.5 per cent of all births (262) in 1999 (Table 4.11). Both reviews of the Maternity and Infant Care Scheme raise questions as to take-up of the scheme and the tendency of some women to avail of private medical care as an alternative.

Looking at statistical patterns regarding women who are potential mothers indicates that between 1971 and 2000, there has been an increase of 366,800 in the core childbearing age group of 15–49 year olds (Table 4.2). Hence more women are potential users of maternity services. This has implications for consumers, policy makers and service providers. The increased hospitalisation and thus management of childbirth has led to an increased dependency on expensive labour-intensive technology. As the numbers of births rise, there is potentially a greater demand for direct maternity and infant care as well as wider social support services. During the 1970 to 2000 period, the number of women giving birth for the first time aged under 25 and over 35 have both decreased, changing the age profile of mothers and shortening the period in which women are likely to give birth to the ten-year period between 25 and 35 years. This also has implications for planners, as research presented in this book demonstrates that women in this age group are less likely to give birth to babies of low birth weight, which places an extra demand on services. During the period 1970 to 2000, the total fertility rate has declined, while at the same time the number of first-time mothers has increased. This has implications for maternity services as first-time mothers are viewed by obstetricians as "an unknown quantity" and thus at higher risk. It also points to a need for greater support services as first-time motherhood is a life-changing experience for women and many might find themselves in need of social support. The number of women having families of four or more children has ·decreased dramatically from 21.8 per cent in 1971 to 4.5 per cent in 2000 (Table 4.6).

One of the most significant changes in terms of outcome of birth is the decline in maternal mortality from 17 per 100,000 in 1971 to 2 in 100,000 in 2000, with a corresponding decline in pre-natal, neonatal and infant mortality. These patterns are important as they are often interpreted as evidence that the increased hospi-talisation of childbirth, as well as higher rates of intervention, have been responsible for this improvement in outcome. This de-bate is further explored later in this book. This analysis of statisti-cal patterns relating to pregnancy and maternity has raised some important issues in terms of social policy, relating not only to health policies but also to welfare and labour market policies and these too are examined in the following chapters.

Chapter Five

ON THE WAY TO THE LABOUR WARD

Chapter Two examined the social and medical models of child-birth by introducing the concepts of language, time, fear, fragmentation, choice, control, dignity, cost, power, place and health and safety. In this and the subsequent two chapters these concepts are interwoven and applied thematically to Irish maternity policies for the 30-year period from 1970 to 2000. The concepts are presented following the natural progression of the stages of pregnancy from conception to lactation, that is, through the maternity period, following the themes of ante-natal care and education, labour and delivery and the postpartum period. This is done to arrive at an understanding of the extent to which Irish maternity policies are or are not woman-centered. In order to achieve this goal, medical research and evidence are presented, drawing largely on the work of Enkin et al. (2000), *A Guide to Effective Care in Pregnancy and Childbirth*, the significance of which was explained in Chapter One.

CHOICES IN EARLY PREGNANCY

From the moment a woman becomes aware that she may be pregnant and wants her suspicions confirmed, she is faced with choices. The choice she makes may depend on her level of education, where she lives and on her socio-economic status. Her choice will also be influenced by the stories and anecdotes about childbirth she has heard while growing up. Currently, in Ireland, a woman who wants to confirm her pregnancy can buy a pregnancy testing kit over the counter in a pharmacy at a cost of between €15 and €25. Interestingly, the 1997 *Report of the Maternity and Infant Care Scheme Review Group* recommends that with reference to diagnosis of pregnancy, the cost of the pregnancy testing kit should be reimbursable as part of the remuneration paid in respect of the scheme (Page 14: Section 2.13). This has not happened.

A woman who can afford to do so can take such a test and do it in the privacy of her own home and cope with the result in whatever way she wishes. She can keep the news to herself for a while or share it with whom she chooses. She may be overwhelmed by the result, either by joy or sorrow, but to a large extent she has the privacy and space in which to deal with the outcome. Another option is for a woman to go to her general practitioner or to a maternity unit and ask for a pregnancy test. If a woman chooses this option, she immediately becomes a medical record, a file and a number, and has entered the public route towards the delivery ward. From the very beginning, women are forced to make choices and are fragmented into different groups. In maternity hospitals, women are asked such questions as their marital status, religion and occupation and are categorised accordingly. These are social issues. Women are asked questions on their general health, their previous pregnancies and age and are then categorised and labelled according to risk. These are health issues. Furthermore, in Ireland women are divided into "public" and "private" patients.

The woman who has taken the test in the privacy of her own home can take time to think, to reflect on her next step, and decide with whom she will share her new status. The woman, one of a very small number in Ireland (Table 4.11), who decides to opt for a home birth will, where possible, choose her midwife and will receive ante-natal care and education in her own home. The midwife will be invited into her home and together they will decide who will attend the birth and where it will occur. From the very beginning, choice and fragmentation are issues. The woman who has entered the hospital system becomes a medical case, a pathogenic case, and becomes fragmented into a body with a womb, blood and urine, breasts and a pelvis. She begins to learn a new, medicalised language. On the other hand, the woman who has not shared her news with the public world of medicine is still a whole person, in control of her own destiny and her own ante-natal decisions.

HEALTH AND SAFETY

Childbirth has always, historically and cross-culturally, been wrapped in a shroud of fear. Pregnancy and childbirth can present dangers for both women and babies. All childbirth practitioners acknowledge this risk. However, emphasis on risk tends to be stressed by those who practice the profession of obstetrics. To quote from *Obstetrics by Ten Teachers*, one of the main obstetric textbooks for students, now in its sixteenth edition:

> Most women in the obstetric scene have no disease and are going through a physiological process. This, however, can alter sharply to pathology and the borderline between the two must be watched carefully (Chamberlain et al., 1995: *xv*).

Success or failure are presented in terms of rates of maternal and perinatal mortality and morbidity. Murphy-Lawless (1998b) questions the accuracy of this reporting system as there is evidence of under-classification and misclassification, in both developed and developing countries, of mortality rates regarding birth outcome. Patterns of progress or of evolution in maternity care are understood in terms of decreases in these statistical trends and patterns. However, quality of care is seldom analysed and women's feelings and emotions are seldom a subject of study. Women are taught to believe that if they leave the highly medicalised, technologised hospital with a healthy baby, and that even though the woman herself may have experienced a variety of interventions and may have been cut and stitched either during an episiotomy or a caesarean section, then she should be grateful. The fact that a woman may have learned that she could not give birth to her own baby but had to be delivered of it, that she could not nurture her own baby for a variety of reasons, is somehow perceived as ir-relevant. It brings to mind Pahl's concept of the "black box". Pahl (1990) refers to the household as a black box, into which income enters one side and exits the other side without any clear analysis of what occurs within this black box, in terms of control, choice, management and distribution. In this instance, the hospital is the black box. A pregnant woman enters one door and a woman with a baby exits the same door some days later. The processes that occur inside in the black box are unmentioned, unanalysed and unaccounted for, despite the fact that the woman who emerges often speaks a new language and uses words, when listened to, which include rape, barbarity, violation, hate, fear, helplessness and anger (as recounted by several women during the *Mother and Child 2000* Conference, 1996, and *Changing Childbirth Now* work-shop, 1997).

RISK PREDICTION

Childbirth involves risk (Murphy-Lawless, 1998a, 1998b). Obstet-rics stresses this risk. The medical model of childbirth is based on the belief that pregnancy is a pathogenic state and that all pregnant women and their babies are potentially at risk. In accordance with this, scales have been developed to predict risk; that is, to predict which women are most likely to need obstetric care and their ba-bies to need emergency care on birth. When women attend for ante-natal care, both at hospital and at home, their risk status is as-sessed. Risk in childbirth is associated with age, parity, social class, obstetric history, previous stillbirth, neonatal death, abortion, cae-sarean section, coexisting disease, hypertension and diabetes. This concept is applied to a woman at her first ante-natal appointment and is the context in which the woman is subsequently assessed as she progresses through the stages of maternity care, from ante-natal to labour and delivery and the post-partum period. Enkin et al. refer to the formal risk prediction system as:

> A mixed blessing for the individual woman and her baby.
> They may help to provide a minimum level of care and atten-

tion in settings where these are inadequate. In other settings, however, formal risk scoring results in a variety of unwarranted interventions. The introduction of risk scoring into clinical practice carries the danger of replacing a potential risk of adverse outcome with the certain risk of dubious treatments and interventions (2000: 52).

ANTE-NATAL CARE

Ante-natal care is generally presented to women as something positive. It can mean different things to different people. Wagner explains that "very little is known about the content of routine prenatal care and its impact on the health of the woman and her baby" (1994: 64). Interestingly, he argues that most research has focused on the behaviour of the mother, rather than on the actions of the providers, which is what is normally studied in health care. He continues: ". . . does a system of routine visits to health care providers during pregnancy improve the chances for a live, healthy baby and mother?" and concedes that "the available evidence indicated that routine prenatal care probably has an overall beneficial effect of some sort, at least for some pregnancies" (1994: 64).

Porter and MacIntyre (1989) examine the psychosocial effects of ante-natal care, questioning whether it meets the needs of women for support, information and encouragement during pregnancy and the puerperium. They summarise women's perceptions of ante-natal care as long waiting hours, discontinuity of care, production-line atmosphere and communication failures. These are issues which have been raised by women in Ireland (Department of Health, 1995, 1997a, 1997b).

Currell (1990) explains that ante-natal care did not develop until the early twentieth century when the first ante-natal clinic was opened in Edinburgh in 1915, and by 1935 it was estimated that about 30 per cent of women were receiving such care. The accepted four-weekly intervals for attendance, from 16 to 36 weeks, and weekly intervals thereafter had become the norm and is still common practice. The 1997 *Report of the Maternity and Infant Care Scheme Review Group*, acknowledging that combined care (that is, care that is shared between general practitioner and maternity unit) is the best and most convenient form of ante-natal care for the majority of mothers, accepts the schedule recommended by the Irish College of General Practitioners and the Institute of Obstetricians and Gynaecologists. The woman carries her own medical record cards between the general practitioner and maternity unit. While a woman should have access to her own maternity records, it is important that these be explained accurately and sensitively to her, as a woman could potentially spend hours agonising over a medical term which she may not understand. The 1997 report claims that it is essential that each woman is seen as early as possible in pregnancy by a medical practitioner and remains under medical and midwifery supervision throughout the ante-natal and post-natal periods. This is a very limited conception of "care" and would be better described as a type of supervision and monitoring. The recommended schedule of visits is outlined in Table 5.1.

Table 5.1 Schedule of Attendance for Ante-natal and Post-natal Care under the Maternity and Infant Care Scheme

Before 12th week of pregnancy — first visit to general practitioner
Before 20th week of pregnancy — first visit to hospital
24 weeks — general practitioner
28 weeks — general practitioner, hospital for first pregnancy
30 weeks — general practitioner
32 weeks — hospital
34 weeks — general practitioner
36 weeks — hospital
37 weeks — general practitioner
38 weeks — hospital
39 weeks — general practitioner
40 weeks — hospital

Source: Department of Health (1997b) *Report of the Review Group of the Maternity and Infant Care Scheme*

In contrast, the woman who chooses to avail of the services of a domiciliary midwife has the option of having all ante-natal care in her own home, at a time that suits, and with her partner and her other children present, if she desires. Ford (2001), in her review of home birth services in Ireland, indicates that the three pilot schemes in progress in the ERHA, the Western Health Board and the Southern Health Board include some ante-natal care in the woman's home.

In practical terms, attending for ante-natal care means 12 appointments, or situations where women have to present themselves either at the maternity unit or general practitioner, arrange child care, transport, time off work, with no assistance from the state. Yet women are led to believe that this is an essential part of pregnancy and that their babies will suffer if the procedure is not followed. Wagner writes that "current prenatal care is designed for the convenience of the people who provide it" (1994: 74). Enkin et al. conclude that:

> Pregnant women may have other priorities besides care, such as finding the time and money to provide for children already in the household. A pregnant woman does not leave her work, community and family responsibilities behind when she steps into the clinic or the doctor's office. . . . Persons providing maternity care share the collective responsibility for ensuring that effective care is not only known, but is also available, accessible and affordable to all women who require it (2000: 17, 22).

The Ante-natal Booking Interview

Ante-natal care begins with the booking interview. Methven (1990: 49) summarises the range of objectives of the ante-natal interview as on a continuum from obtaining and recording information, establishing risk, booking a bed for confinement, to establishing a relationship with the carer and discussing expectations in relation to childbirth and the post-natal period and to plan accordingly:

The booking interview opens the case notes, which will become a permanent record of the mother's progress and the
development of her baby . . . [the interview] can provide a forum for dialogue, information giving and an opportunity to
initiate parent craft education where this is appropriate
(Methven, 1990: 50).

NEW TECHNOLOGY: THE BIRTH MACHINE

Marsden Wagner refers to:

The birth machine; a wide array of medical interventions, often of a technical nature, used before, during and following
birth. . . . The birth machine has become a centre of controversy because it unites two key issues in the evolution of
health care: birth as a health promoting act and the role of
technology in appropriate health care (1994: 8).

Pursuing the Birth Machine, written by Wagner, is based on a
World Health Organisation (WHO) evaluation of the cost, efficacy
and risk of the expanding "birth machine". The WHO undertook
to stage a number of international, interdisciplinary meetings designed to bring a scientific and multidisciplinary approach to the
task of identifying the best ways of ensuring the safest outcome
for women and babies during pregnancy, birth and following
birth. "We reminded ourselves that women are not just ambula-
tory incubators and intermittent milk factories" (Wagner, 1994:
58).

Looking at ante-natal care in Ireland since the 1970s demonstrates the increasing power and momentum of the birth machine
in Irish maternity units. Interventions are becoming more common, more regular and more expected. Traditionally, maternal
and fetal assessment involved conversation, touch and weighing.
Modern interventions include amniocentesis, chorionic villus
sampling (CVS) and ultrasound scanning. It is beyond the scope
of this book to examine each of these procedures in detail; however an examination of the preponderance of ultrasound scanning
in ante-natal care in Ireland is presented.

Ultrasound Scan (USS)

> The casual observer might be forgiven for wondering why the
> medical profession is now involved in the wholesale examina-
> tion of pregnant women using machines emanating vastly dif-
> ferent powers of energy which is not proven to be of any
> clinical value by operators who are not certified as competent
> to perform the examinations (Meire, 1987: 1122).

Looking at patterns in Irish maternity hospitals, ultrasound scanning (USS) has, since the 1970s, become an important feature of
ante-natal appointments. This is despite the questions still loom-
ing regarding the long-term effects of the scan on the developing
fetus. In the Rotunda at the end of the first full year of the availability of ultrasound scanning, the 1979 clinical report states that
"there is still, I feel, too much reliance placed on ultrasound reports to the exclusion of clinical assessment, especially by younger
staff members" (page 62). In 1982, the clinical report of the Rotunda states:

> Ultrasound continues as a vital part of ante-natal care. This
> year it has been the policy to scan every first visit attending
> the hospital. It is hoped in the near future to re-scan the nor-
> mal patients routinely at 28-30 weeks gestation, thereby ensur-
> ing at least 2 scans per patient during the ante-natal care (page
> 62).

In 1983, the clinical report stated: " . . . the number of scans performed continues to soar".

Meanwhile, in the National Maternity Hospital, in 1981:

> . . . it was disappointing to find that only 60 per cent of babies
> were born within one week of the ultrasound expected date of
> delivery, although 90 per cent were born within two weeks of
> this date (page 83).

Despite this, in 1992, 11 years later, 57 per cent of scans were undertaken to estimate expected date of delivery (EDD). In 1983, "it
is perhaps worth mentioning that it has never been our policy to
perform routine ultrasound scans . . . we are still not in a position

to state that ultrasound is absolutely without risk to the developing fetus" (page 81). Despite this statement, a policy decision was made in that year to scan late pregnancies.

In 1984, the Diagnostic Methods Committee of the British Institute of Radiology examined the evidence regarding diagnostic ultrasound. They recommended that ultrasound scans should only be used for a valid medical reason and they made recommendations regarding the output of scanning machines and the training of personnel (Wells, 1987a, 1987b). In the National Maternity Hospital in 1992:

> The biggest increase over the previous year was in scans done at the patient's request for reassurance . . . the hospital policy is to offer a scan to confirm dates (1992: 100).

This is in line with Proud's observation:

> Most pregnant women expect to have an ultrasound scan. For many indeed it is an integral part of having a baby. They look forward to it and so, often, do their partners. This privileged look at the baby may be anticipated by both parents with great excitement. . . . A degree of bonding takes place as a result of the scan (Proud, 1990: 114).

How did women traditionally bond with their unborn babies? Proud (1990) outlines how the use of USS has become common practice in ante-natal care, that women now expect it and that many women feel deprived if not offered a scan. In 1994, the clinical report of the National Maternity Hospital stated that "patient demands and expectations of ultrasound continue to increase and guidelines for the rational use of ultrasound were drawn up and gradually implemented" (1994: 59). Proud queries the use of ultrasound:

> Ultrasounds cannot provide a solution to every diagnostic problem and in some instances other resources may be more appropriately used. Conversely, the full potential of ultrasound may not always be realised (1990: 105).

Questions have been raised as to the possible effects of ultrasound.

Wagner (1994: 83) indicates the emergence in some countries of commercial scanning offering "baby-book" and "fun-ultrasound" to produce photographs and videos. These are now available in maternity units in Northern Ireland. He states that "it is essential to make the distinction between its selective use for specific indications and for its routine use as a screening procedure" (1994: 83). Wells echoes this in his research on the use of ultrasound scanning:

> The prudent use of ultrasound diagnosis depends on it being used cautiously, carefully, circumspectly, judiciously, sensibly and wisely. Like other technologies in medicine diagnostic ultrasound is a resource, which should be used with skill and good judgement (1987a: 392).

It is clear that routine scanning has become the norm in the large maternity units in Ireland. Proud indicates the likelihood of such screening procedures to increase a woman's stress:

> During ultrasound investigations and other screening procedures performed in the ante-natal period . . . parents are subjected to a great deal of stress (Proud: 1990: 108).

This is echoed by Tew, who claims:

> The first results will give most women the reassurance they hope for, but for some they will be equivocal and indicate the need for further tests, which generate further anxiety, while for the small minority they will confirm the woman's worst fears, leaving her to make very difficult decisions (1995: 130).

As regards the effects of scanning on the fetus, research has begun. So far, conflicting results are emerging that point to the need for further research, which will take into account the frequency of scanning, the expertise of the technician, the strength of the scan and other variables. However, there appears to be some evidence to indicate there may be a link between ultrasound scans and dyslexia and problems of delayed speech. Beech and Robinson (1994), Wagner (1994) and Tew (1995) review this literature. Problems of intra-uterine growth retardation as a result of routine ultrasound scanning have also been raised (Beech and Robinson, 1994). Enkin et al., reviewing literature on ultrasound scanning, conclude that:

> The value of the selective ultrasound for specific indications in pregnancy has been clearly established. The place, if any, for routine ultrasound has not been determined as yet (2000: 58).

Low Birth Weight and Ante-natal Care

Irish women do attend for ante-natal care; for example 66.9 per cent of women availed of ante-natal care under the Maternity and Infant Care Scheme in 1997. Wagner indicates that the social aspects of good health are seldom addressed in ante-natal care. Issues like nutrition, smoking and alcohol consumption are paid cursory attention. Yet there is a heavy concentration on medical aspects of pregnancy. He looks at the issue of birth weight and how in western societies the prevention of low birth weight is seen as a goal of ante-natal care (1994: 68).

As perinatal mortality has decreased, the survival rate of low birth weight babies has increased, raising questions about morbidity patterns. Infant birth weight is one of the most important determinants of health and survival after birth (O'Campo et al., 1995: 279). A baby is classified as being of low birth weight if it weighs less than 2,500 grams; less than 1,500 grams is a very low birth weight (VLBW); and those less than 1,000 grams are extremely very low birth weight (EVLBW). Chamberlain et al. (1995) show that there has been a huge reduction in neonatal mortality in the past 20 years. In Ireland neonatal mortality has decreased from 12.2 per 1,000 live births in 1971 to 4 per 1,000 live births in 2000 (Table 4.19). Only about 1–2 per cent of newborn babies require intensive care. Low birth weight babies are more likely to experience respiratory distress syndrome (RDS), bronchopulmonary dysplasia (BDP) and intraventricular haemorrhage (IVH): "As such, the LBW preterm offers a prototype of the biologically high risk child" (McCarton et al., 1995: 330). Short-term problems for babies of low birth weight include lower respiratory tract infection, while long-term problems include neurodevelopmental conditions, learning disorders and perhaps behavioural problems.

Kitzinger (1995) outlines some of the more common causes of low birth weight. Intra Uterine Growth Retardation (IUGR) is often associated with smoking in pregnancy. Nicotine constricts blood vessels, thus affecting the blood flow through the placenta. IURG is also caused by carbon monoxide and thyocinate in cigarette smoke; therefore passive smoking is an issue for pregnant women. Maternal smoking is one of the most important risk factors that is avoidable: "Maternal smoking decreases infant birth weight on average by 200 grams, primarily by retarding fetal growth after the 30th week of pregnancy" (McCarton et al., 1995: 280). There is some evidence that this could be linked to maternal nutrition, in that the woman who smokes is likely to eat less. Low birth weight is also associated with alcohol abuse and violence against the pregnant woman. Newberger et al. (1992) indicate a link between abuse and abdominal trauma, placental damage, uterine contractions, premature rupture of the membranes, infection related to forced sex, and exacerbating already existing factors, for example, hypertension and diabetes, stress, smoking and diet. Kitzinger (1997) explores the very sensitive issue of sexual abuse and childbirth.

For some babies, birth weight is appropriate for gestation (Tew, 1995: 120); for others not so. Many of the causes of premature birth are similar to those for retarded growth. These include maternal stress and inadequate diet. Some babies are low birth weight because of genetic factors; others are full-term and have low birth weight, while others are born prematurely and so the gestation period was shorter than the average. Thus, low birth weight is associated with prematurity, intra-uterine retarded growth or both.

Medical intervention has had little success (Creasy, 1991) in preventing low birth weight. However, social interventions have led to success. Social interventions which have been found to have relevance to birth weight include smoking, stress and nutrition (Wagner, 1994: 69). Wagner indicates that ante-natal care has tended to focus on the medical rather than the social causes of low birth weight: ". . . the damage done by poverty to pregnancy and birth must be countered by social and financial solutions and not more medical attention" (Wagner, 1994: 73). He continues:

> Routine pre-natal ultrasound scans will not counteract the effects of chronic malnutrition; social solutions such as ensuring a good system of emotional support from relatives and friends to pregnant women, may soften some of the impact of poverty (Wagner, 1994: 75).

Chamberlain et al. (1995) indicate that younger mothers tend to have smaller babies and that the heaviest children tend to be born when the mother's age is between 25 and 30 years. This is very significant for Ireland, for in Chapter Four (Table 4.5) it was demonstrated that Irish women now tend to have their first babies in the ten years between age 25 and 35; therefore, these mothers have a greater chance of heavier and thus healthier babies.

ANTE-NATAL EDUCATION

> Ante-natal care operates as a means of social control over women (Mason, 1994: 9).

While women are becoming socialised and medicalised in ante-natal care in Ireland, they are simultaneously being socialised into the role of pregnant woman and mother in ante-natal education. Mason (1995) indicates how the increased medicalisation of pregnancy and maternity has led to the increased prevalence of childbirth education: ante-natal classes, parentcraft classes, mothercraft classes and preparation for labour and relaxation classes have "become an intrinsic part of what is generally recognised as ante-natal care in the Western world today" (Mason, 1995: 1). It is to this that we will now turn our attention.

Oakley (1979) describes the historical development of the natural childbirth philosophy, associated with such names as

Dick-Read (1942), Leboyer (1975) and Odent (1984). This can be seen as synonymous with the development of childbirth education.

> None of these prescriptions for natural childbirth places women as people at the centre of their own experience of childbirth (Oakley, 1979: 22).

Kitzinger, an experienced childbirth educator, midwife, anthropologist, mother and grandmother, acknowledges the role of ante-natal education in the context of lifelong family patterns (1995: 16). She views childbirth education as having a role in preparing parents not only for childbirth but also for lifelong parenthood. She says it should involve passing on information and developing self-confidence.

Williams and Booth (1984: 3–4), in one of the classic textbooks on childbirth education, identify the aims of ante-natal education as:

- To build up a woman's confidence in herself "and in those who are looking after her"

- To ensure a healthy and happy pregnancy; "happy in looking forward with joyful anticipation . . . to the birth"

- To be prepared for labour so as to achieve satisfaction "within the context of safe maternity care"

- To promote the airing of problems

- To prepare women for the physical and emotional care of the baby.

As Oakley states, "A revision is needed of the goals and content of ante-natal education as it is offered to pregnant women today" (1980: 282). Mason outlines the development of ante-natal care in Irish maternity units, recognising as a practising childbirth educator herself that "the manner in which ante-natal classes are conducted can have a profound effect on women's perceptions of how they might experience birth and on the effectiveness of ante-natal education" (1994: 3). Referring to "childbirth education" as consisting of two strands — midwife-led and physiotherapist-led education — Mason indicates how ante-natal classes were introduced into the major maternity hospitals in Dublin by physiotherapists and how gradually midwives began to become involved, leading to the development of integrated classes from the 1970s onwards (1995: 5). She indicates that while the ante-natal classes in Irish maternity units run by physiotherapists concentrate on preparation, the midwives concentrate on parentcraft. They overlap in the area of pain relief and in the process of labour itself "which may or may not cause some professional disagreement" (1995: 6).

Neeson (1995), in her review of services provided in Irish maternity units, points out that ante-natal classes are organised at times unsuitable to women employed in the paid labour market and also militate against mothers who have childcare responsibilities and cannot attend due to childcare commitments. The timing of classes also militates against involvement of partners who may be in paid employment and so unable to attend during regular working hours. In fact, some maternity units do not allow partners to attend all classes. There is also a question of economic access, as some classes charge a fee while others do not. While there is a case for women attending classes in the unit in which they will deliver, for reasons of preparation and familiarity, there is also a case for women attending classes in the area in which they live so as to make contact with other expectant mothers with a view to post-natal support. However, physiotherapists providing classes outside the hospital scheme charge fees of around €90, which again excludes a wide number of prospective parents. Ante-natal classes which use yoga, meditation and other techniques generally classified as alternative practices, are also available but again only to women with the resources to attend. Many women who attend the alternative classes suggest they chose this route having attended hospital-based classes previously and being dissatisfied with the focus of those classes on risk and on what could go wrong. Others indicated dissatisfaction with policies that deter partners from attending classes. Here again, women are fragmented by socio-economic status, education, geography, childcare and work responsibilities.

Wiley and Merriman (1996) conducted a survey of women's health needs, drawing from a national sample of women aged between 18 and 60 years. Drawn from the register of electors, the multi-stage random sample involved interviews with 2,988 women. Wiley and Merriman equate the growth in ante-natal education with the move from home to hospital "to prepare expectant mothers for the less familiar hospital environment" (1996: 97). Their findings indicate that close to 31 per cent of mothers attend ante-natal classes in preparation for childbirth. Those who did not attend ante-natal classes gave the following reasons: there were none available at the time, classes were too far away, they were not of any use, they had done them before or had no time. The 1996 study indicated a lower rate of attendance at ante-natal classes for medical card holders and younger women. Attendance at ante-natal education classes increased in relation to level of education generally. Kennedy and Murphy-Lawless (2002) present evidence that indicates there is a very poor attendance at ante-natal classes for asylum-seeking women in Ireland. This is further discussed in Chapter Eight.

THE DELIVERY SUITE

> They lie like stranded whales, enormous undulations of flesh, immobilised and trapped on narrow tables under glaring lights. Each of the four women is separated from the next by only a curtain. From between her legs a wire projects. It is linked to a machine with a rapidly flashing green eye, and from this a long strip of ticker-tape is steadily but tidily vomited, falling in thickening folds as time wears on. Another wire, recording uterine pressure, connects with the machine too and produces its own eruption of jagged lines. "Lie still", the women are told. "Any movement will interfere with the print-out of the monitor." But it is not possible for them to move. Each has no sensation at all from above her belly to be-

low her feet. Taped to one shoulder is the epidural catheter
through which more anaesthetic can be injected when the feeling returns (Kitzinger, in Foreword to Odent, 1984: xiv).

The birth machine begins to roll as the expectant woman tests her
urine to detect certain oestrogens, which indicate pregnancy. This
machine continues to roll through the radiology units of the out-
patients department, and gathers momentum as the first signs of
labour are acknowledged; or perhaps, the corollary, there are no
signs of labour, but the birth mechanics had predicted an expected date of delivery which has come and gone so it is time to
intervene and to deliver the baby from the mother.

Chapter Six

THE BIRTH

A closer examination of patterns in Irish maternity units will illustrate the increase in medical interventions in childbirth in Ireland since 1970. This book draws on statistical data from the clinical reports of the three major Maternity Hospitals in Dublin, the National Maternity Hospital (Holles Street), the Rotunda and the Coombe Women's Hospital (formerly the Coombe Lying-In Hospital). Since the late 1980s, more than one-third of Irish women give birth annually in these hospitals (Table 4.13). They are hospitals to which women from all over Ireland can be referred for specialist care. These hospitals are important as they are also training hospitals for medical students from the Irish College of Surgeons, University College Dublin, Trinity College Dublin, for midwives and general nurses as well as for General Practitioners taking their Higher Diplomas in Obstetrics and Gynaecology, for social workers and for physiotherapists. The importance of the three main maternity hospitals in Dublin is therefore apparent from the large number of births that take place each year within their walls and for their extensive role in training and thereby influencing generations of health professionals.

Since 1976, Comhairle na nOspidéal official policy in Ireland is that all births should take place in an obstetric-staffed maternity unit. The 1976 discussion document *Development of Hospital Maternity Services* recommended that:

> If the basic aims of ensuring delivery and giving the infant the best chance of optimal health and normal development are to

be achieved, every expectant mother should have ready access
to care at a consultant-staffed obstetric neonatal unit (1976: 12).

While this recommendation is that all women should have "access",
this was in fact explained as "the implementation of the recommendations in this document would involve the closing of existing small
maternity units, which are not viable, and fall below the existing
standards for the practice of modern obstetrics" (1976: 13).

This was the death knell which heralded the closure of the
smaller maternity units in Ireland in subsequent years. Looking at
statistics for the size of maternity units in 1978 (Table 4.12), 19.8
per cent of births took place in maternity units with fewer than
1,000 births per annum (average fewer than three births in 24
hours). By 1983 the figure had dropped to 11.3 per cent and to 5.5
per cent in 1993. Figures are not available after 1993.

PLACE OF BIRTH

Barry (1992: 11) argues that in the 1970s in Ireland the issue for
women was contraceptive rights while in the 1980s the issue was
abortion rights. It would seem justified to claim that the 1990s saw
the beginning of a wave of discontent and questioning slowly rising over the issue of birth rights, or more explicitly women having
choice and control in the area of childbirth. This wave had
emerged in the 1980s with a number of groups, including Cuidiú
(the Irish Childbirth Trust), Irish Association for Improvements in
Maternity Services and the Home Birth Centre.

Home Births: The Evidence

The Home Birth Centre (known since 1997 as the Home Birth Association) has very clear aims and objectives which include increasing
public awareness of birth as a natural event rather than as a medical problem and presenting home birth as a viable option; working
towards the reintegration of domiciliary births into the general maternity service; and informing and advising parents on various aspects of organising a home birth while stressing that all home

births should be attended by qualified medical personnel as far as is practicable. The Association, without any funding from the Department of Health (which consistently refuses to support the Association, stating that the Department's policy is that all births should take place in obstetric-staffed maternity units), provides practical support and assistance to parents who choose a home birth, advises parents on their legal rights to have a home birth and, in particular, informs them of the Health Board's statutory obligations to provide them with medical and midwifery services.

There had developed in Ireland, as in other countries (Tew, 1995), a division between those advocating domiciliary births — usually midwives and voluntary pressure groups — and medical practitioners — generally, male obstetricians — advocating hospital births and vehemently refuting the safety of home births. In response to this, an Eastern Health Board committee was established to look at the issue of domiciliary births in Ireland. While the committee did draw on the services of a range of professionals, it consisted totally of medical doctors. This brings to mind the words of Wagner, who describes how policy-makers formulate policy on perinatal care, whilst knowing little about the area; they:

> . . . usually organise some kind of expert advisory committee by turning to a university medical school and perhaps obstetrical and paediatric organisations. The expert committee thus formed usually consists of several professors of obstetrics and paediatrics and possibly one or two public health physicians. As a result, the advice they give (usually behind closed doors) is based only on the medical model (1994: 4).

From the very outset, the 1983 report treats flippantly the home birth movement, describing it as:

> . . . a number of women who have not found hospital-based childbirth a rewarding experience have set up an organisation called the Home Birth Centre of Ireland. The aim of the centre is to foster domiciliary births in suitable cases (Foreword).

Yet the Home Birth Centre is an organisation which is very clear about its objectives and its constitution (Dunlop, 1998).

While the 1983 Eastern Health Board report rejects outright domiciliary births, it advocates a more woman-centred service, proposing smaller, more user-friendly units. However, an examination of size of maternity units in relation to number of births would indicate that the opposite has in fact occurred (Table 4.12), and this for reasons of improving the control and workings of the birth machine. Figures for length of stay in hospital, post-delivery, are important, as many policy documents advocating the importance of hospital births argue that hospitals could be made more user-friendly if the length of stay were shortened. These statistics show that for the majority of women delivering a single child, the length of stay would appear to be around five days. However, these figures are misleading as they refer to the average overall figure and thus include problem births. Consultation with the three maternity units in Dublin indicates that their policies allow a first-time mother in a public ward two nights in hospital and for a caesarean birth the length of stay is a maximum of seven days. This, they explain, is dictated by the number of available beds and VHI regulations rather than maternal requirements. It also depends on the number of patients in the hospital at the time.

In 1989, the Department of Health (1989) *Report of the Commission on Health Funding*, which incidentally was chaired by a mother, Dr Miriam Hederman O'Brien, stated:

> We regard the Domiciliary Maternity Scheme as an important element in preventative care for mothers and infants which might be used less if a charge was imposed on those currently eligible for it. Although maternity care is largely provided in acute hospitals, attendance as an out-patient for ante- and post-natal care is not a practical proposition for many mothers. The maximum saving to the State of requiring the present Category to pay for free general practitioner care during pregnancy would be less than one million pounds (*Report of the Commission on Health Funding*, 1989: 222, section 11.58).

Furthermore, it states as a recommendation that "all persons should have entitlement to the Domiciliary Maternity Scheme as a core service". However, four years later, the Second Commission on the Status of Women accepts the status quo — the hospitalisation of childbirth — while calling for improvements in services. It stresses the importance of practices and facilities in maternity hospitals, reflecting the needs and wishes of the women who use them (1993: 340).

> The lack of single delivery units, for example, in some maternity hospitals can cause unnecessary distress to women, particularly first time mothers, if they are involuntarily observers at other births . . . the health and well being of new mothers and their children should be based on a recognition of the needs of patients in a wider context, for example, adopting a flexible approach to visiting times by immediate relatives, providing advice and support with regard to breast feeding. . . . It is important that maternity hospitals and units should take account of women's experiences as users of the system.

The Commission report reinforced a concept of rights in relation to employment and the public sphere in general, but this did not extend to the reproductive sphere.

Department of Health policy that childbirth should occur in obstetric-staffed maternity units was reiterated in 1995 in *Developing a Policy for Women's Health*, the discussion document on women's health which failed to take on board the research which shows that for the majority of women, those not in the high risk group, home is a safe place in which to give birth (Wagner, 1994; MacFarlane and Campbell, 1994; Tew, 1995). The 1995 Department of Health report states:

> It is sometimes argued that there should be greater support for home births from the health services. While recognising that mothers who choose to give birth in their own home are entitled to the medical and midwifery care they require, there are good arguments why the health services should discourage home births. The main reason is because the health of the new born child is at greater risk in the home than in a well staffed and equipped maternity unit (1995: 35).

This is a very strong statement and I would regard it as potentially scare-mongering. It refers vaguely to "good arguments" without reference or elaboration and claims that the newborn child is at greater risk at home while again it does not document any research to substantiate this. It continues:

> There is a clear need for maternity hospitals to respect the unique experience of each mother and father by giving parents as much choice as possible and by simulating a domestic environment for those with a normal delivery and labour (1995: 3–4).

This statement denies the seriousness and importance of the whole domiciliary/hospital birth debate by simplifying the argument to one of physical surroundings. It reduces the debate to the traditional unsubstantiated argument which associates the decline in mortality with an increase in the hospitalisation of birth:

> The perinatal mortality rate fell from 24 per 1,000 in 1970 to less than 10 per 1,000 live and still births between 1970 and 1990. Maternal mortality is now below the EU average and is currently two per 100,000 live and stillbirths. This improvement can be attributed to good ante-natal and perinatal care provided by our hospitals. Many of the criticisms of services which encourage women to give birth at home would be met if the maternity units could further facilitate women giving birth by providing domestic style surroundings with more choice, the minimum of unnecessary interference as well as early discharge home after birth (1995: 35).

Midwifery in Ireland

The 1995 Department of Health Report joins the backlash against midwives who have traditionally supported mothers through the birth process and have now become relegated to obstetric assistants, by emphasising the responsibility of midwives to empathise with the women for whom they care:

> Midwives, as the profession which is responsible for the care of women in normal labour and childbirth, have a particular

responsibility to recognise the changing aspirations of women
in relation to childbirth and to facilitate an appropriate response to that change (1995: 35).

This statement does not acknowledge the importance of midwives
historically and internationally, as outlined by Donnison (1977,
1988), Murphy-Lawless (1991a, 1991b) and Tew (1995). The traditional role of midwives was, as the medieval derivation of their
name denotes, to be "with woman" throughout her labour, giving
her emotional support and encouragement. The midwife's skills
lay in ensuring the necessary hygiene and in knowing how to help
the labouring woman to use her own reproductive powers to
bring forth her child naturally and without damage (Tew, 1995: 9).

Traditionally there was no direct entry midwifery training in
Ireland. The Report of the Commission on Nursing (1998) acknowledged this void and recommended the establishment of a
Direct Entry Midwifery Diploma to develop into a Degree in 2002.
This thinking is in line with a 1980 European Directive on Midwives (80/155/EEC) which recommends that direct entry training
should be an option, the role of the midwife in the community as
practitioner, educator and counsellor should be enhanced and refresher courses should be mandatory. The Home Birth Association refers to the value of direct midwifery training in that "the
direct entry system ensures that a midwife's main focus is on birth
as a normal life event rather than a disease or malfunction"
(Home Birth Association leaflet entitled *Midwifery Training and
Practice in Ireland*). Currently in Ireland, midwifery training takes
place in maternity units, so midwives have no opportunity to
learn to deliver babies in a domiciliary setting. As a result of this
training policy, any independent midwives practising in Ireland
have either trained abroad or trained in Ireland in earlier decades.
The decline in domiciliary births can to some extent be explained
by this pattern (O'Connor, 1995). Choice for women is limited, as
those who want to practice domiciliary midwifery are denied access to training in this country while, on the other hand, those
women who wish to have home births do not have the choice.

Within Irish hospitals, there are seven midwifery training schools. Each midwifery student will have completed three years general nursing training. Midwifery training takes two years. This training consists of ante-natal (12 weeks) and intra-natal care (18 weeks) which deals with labour and delivery. The interim report from the Commission on Nursing (An Bord Altranais, 1997: 21) defines a midwife as:

> ... a person who, having been admitted to a midwifery educational programme, duly recognised in the country in which it is located, has successfully completed the prescribed course of studies in midwifery and has acquired the requisite qualifications to be registered and/or legally licensed to practice midwifery. She must be able to give the necessary supervision, care and advice to women during pregnancy, labour and postpartum period, to conduct deliveries on her own responsibility and to care for the newborn and the infant. This care includes preventative measures, the detection of abnormal conditions in mother and child, the procurement of medical assistance and the execution of emergency measures in the absence of medical help. She has an important task in health counselling and education, not only for the women, but also within the family and the community. The work should involve ante-natal education and preparation for parenthood and extends to certain areas of gynaecology, family planning and child care. She may practice in hospitals, clinics, health units, domiciliary conditions or in any other service.

In 1996, the number of midwives registered as active with An Bord Altranais (the Nursing Board) numbered 12,136. The 1997 interim report of the Nursing Commission indicates that many midwives feel that they are becoming de-skilled because of the medicalisation of the childbirth process and that they had been turned into "obstetric nurses rather than the independent practitioners allowed by their education" (1997: 21). This is echoed in the final report of the Commission (1998). It continues to emphasise the importance of midwifery in "the development of a woman-centred service, before, during and after pregnancy". At present there are only 14 practising domiciliary midwives in Ireland and none in some areas of the country.

The status of midwives in Ireland as independent practitioners is very vulnerable. This became visible in 1996 when a complaint was made to An Bord Altranais against Ann O'Ceallaigh, an independent domiciliary midwife, by a senior obstetrician in one of the maternity units under study in this book. Ann O'Ceallaigh refuted the complaint and insisted on expert evidence to refute it, as she felt it was without substance. The Ann O'Ceallaigh Support Group has publicised some facts that have been established which are very significant in terms of women's autonomy both as mothers and as providers of midwifery services. It was not suggested that either the mother or child who were subject to the complaint suffered any ill health after the birth. The mother in question never complained and in fact wrote to the hospital asking that the complaint be dropped. The complaint was in connection with the referral of the mother to hospital at a time judged by the complainant to be too late and to have therefore potentially risked the life and health of the mother. During the lengthy hearings and court actions entailed in this case, Ann O'Ceallaigh called on international experts who reviewed events and came to radically different conclusions about the complainant's interpretation of events.

The Ann O'Ceallaigh case raised major issues in relation to midwifery in Ireland but also in relation to women's autonomy as mothers and as recipients of care. It highlighted the existence of tensions between providers of maternity services based on a medical as opposed to a social model of care. The events that unfolded since 1996 resonate with the sort of events that have historically been associated with the demise of midwifery (Donnison, 1977, 1988).

Following the publication of the 1995 discussion document *Developing a Policy for Women's Health*, extensive consultation took place with women throughout Ireland to discuss their requirements regarding future health policy. Many groups, and particularly those from the Southern Health Board region, where there is a high incidence of unplanned home births because of distance from maternity units and lack of access to domiciliary services, challenged the ethos of the report regarding hospital-based childbirth, urging the Department of Health to consult literature on safety associated with place of birth, and made demands for a more varied range of services. The *Plan for Women's Health* states that "the case for greater support for women who choose to give birth at home was also forcibly made" (1997b: 35) and to meet these demands accepts the recommendations of the 1997 Maternity and Infant Care Review Group.

The Report of the Review Group states that "it is difficult to assess the true demand for births at home because of the absence of domiciliary services on a nation-wide basis". However, in their 1996 survey of women's health, Wiley and Merriman had no such difficulty. They found in their sample that 5 per cent of women gave birth at home intentionally, while 14 per cent of those who did not give birth at home would have liked to have done so. Therefore, nearly 20 per cent of women surveyed were interested in availing of domiciliary services.

The 1997 Department of Health report stresses that the underlying objective of the Maternity and Infant Care Scheme continues to be a safe outcome of a live and healthy mother and baby, and a satisfied and happy family unit (1997b: 21). It refers to women seeking home births as evidence of "the desire on the part of a woman for a positive experience of birth in friendly familiar surroundings where she retains full control of her environment, her body and all procedures" (1997b: 21). They acknowledge that some women may have had previous negative experiences of childbirth which may have been due to "the woman's perception of an unfriendly atmosphere", unwillingness of hospital personnel to provide information "regarding many aspects of pregnancy", procedures carried out without adequate and informed consent, removal of her dignity and autonomy. In response, it recommended that pilot programmes be established and evaluated by the regional Health Boards. It referred to some possible types of provision:

- *Home Environment in a Maternity Hospital*, which is described as "a homely non-clinical environment where the mother would have freedom to move around and her partner and children would be welcome" (1997b: 21). Hospital support would be available for emergencies and the woman and baby would spend a very limited period in hospital.

- *Modified Domino Approach*, which would allow for the midwife and/or GP to attend the woman ante-natally in the community and to be with her in hospital and to attend her post-natally in the community, which would facilitate continuity of care. Again the time spent in hospital would be limited.

The Report states that despite these recommendations "there would continue to be a small number of women who, regardless of policy or professional advice, would insist on having a home birth" (1997b: 230). This patronising attitude places more pressure on the women struggling to exercise their statutory rights to obtain services. They are often made to feel selfish and that they are putting the life of their unborn child at risk (O'Connor, 1995). This is despite the findings of O'Connor's study which indicates that women who have planned domiciliary births are more likely to be educated to a higher standard, which would raise questions around informed choice. The debate which surrounds the safety of domiciliary births is presented later in this chapter.

To cater for women who cannot be persuaded to deliver in or at a maternity hospital/unit, the Review Group recommended that each health board community care management put in place arrangements with the local maternity hospital/unit to provide for a midwife to attend such home birth, claiming that "such an arrangement would ensure the availability of trained experienced midwives and the availability of hospital back-up in the event of an emergency". While acknowledging the lack of midwives trained in domiciliary births, it looks to meet this deficit through recruiting GPs with experience of domiciliary birth, therefore negating the profession of midwifery and deferring to general practitioners who have little training in midwifery either at home or in hospital. It would appear to be more concerned with the fact that "general practitioners may find it difficult to secure medical indemnity insurance to cover attendance on home births" (1997b: 20).

The Expert Group on Domiciliary Births was established in 1997. Its terms of reference were:

- To draw up procedures and protocols for immediate application to the present arrangements for domiciliary births, particularly to legal safeguards

- To suggest locations for pilot schemes in respect of a hospital outreach service and Community Midwives Scheme to draw up protocols for this and assess their outcomes

- Arising from the outcomes of the pilot schemes, make recommendations on the long-term approach and whatever procedures and protocols will be necessary.

As a result of the Expert Group on Domiciliary Births, a pilot scheme came into being in the National Maternity Hospital in 1999. This was a combined Domino and Hospital Outreach Service. The Review of the project, which was published in 2001 by the Women's Health Unit of the ERHA, claims that two of its achievements included providing continuity of care and good interpersonal relationships between clients and midwives and stresses that "there are high levels of personal and professional satisfaction among midwives working in the project" (2001: 25).

In 1997, the Expert Group wrote to each health board requesting them to submit a proposal for pilot projects. In that same year, one woman who exercised her legal right to demand domiciliary services had to resort to employing a solicitor to approach the South Eastern Health Board on her behalf after she herself had made several unsuccessful approaches to the Health Board. As a result, two public health nurses were given special training (which did not involve attending a domiciliary birth but involved watching a video of same), were released from their usual place of work, replaced in that hospital, and accommodated in lodgings for a period of three months. This cost an estimated €64,000. The woman in question, with the two midwives in attendance, gave birth to a healthy baby, which the mother herself attributed at least in part to the fact that she had already given birth to three children, two at home with an experienced domiciliary midwife, and thus felt that she could support and guide her attending midwives through the process (reported at the Home Birth Association Annual Conference 1998 by the mother). Dempsey and Mulcahy (1998), the midwives who attended the birth, have written a report on the project. They recommend that the project should be continued, that the domiciliary midwifery service should remain with the Public Health Nursing Service and that public health nurses providing the service should have had recent midwifery experience. They recommend that regular theoretical and practice refresher courses, with a midwifery component, are necessary, as is additional study leave. The 1998 report is an important milestone in Irish maternity policy as it is the first time that any official report has acknowledged that there exists "evidence from the literature that it is as safe for most women to give birth at home as in hospital" (Dempsey and Mulcahy, 1998: 33).

The Report of the Review Group endorses the views of the Institute of Obstetricians and Gynaecologists and the Royal College of Gynaecologists that "the best place for deliveries is where full emergency services are immediately available and accessible" (1997b: 18). Accessible and available does not mean that the birth should take place in hospital. There are other options: for example, the development of flying squad emergency services. The Report of the Review Group refers to the Comhairle na nOspidéal report of 1976 and the UNICEF report *State of the World's Children* which indicates Ireland's low maternal mortality rate, assuming that there is a correlation between it and place of birth. It ignores evidence to the contrary (1997b: 18). Enkin at al. argue that:

> . . . maternal and perinatal mortality are so low in low risk pregnancies that these cannot be the primary outcome measures for a trial. Yet they are the outcomes of real interest and the source of the polarized concerns. A study looking at issues of less importance would not provide data that are relevant to

those who wish to make a choice based on considerations of safety (2000: 250–251).

The Report of the Review Group states that "in order to reduce the risk of a woman undergoing a bad or negative experience while in hospital, which may impact on the level of demand for births at home", the Patient's Charter should be adhered to, a charter for pregnant women should be introduced and that "an assurance of a friendly atmosphere in hospitals where the dignity and autonomy of the mother is respected" (1997b: 19) should be developed. It further recommends that there should be openness in relation to information giving, flexibility regarding length of stay and "crèche facilities for older children at maternity clinics" (1997b: 19). It recommends "the provision of hot meals to mothers who choose to avail of them following delivery" (1997b: 19). Research by Kennedy and Murphy-Lawless demonstrates that those aspirations had not become a reality as late as 2000 (Kennedy and Murphy-Lawless, 2002).

Referring to women's experiences of childbirth in maternity units in Ireland, the 1997 report states "the mother's voice is sometimes lost in the organised hospital situation" (1997b: 28). To improve the service they recommend the preparation of birthplans prior to hospitalisation, that woman's permission must be given to participate in research or clinical trials, that mothers should be required to give consent for intervention and have the right to refuse interventions. It states, "the use of technology should take place only with the full informed consent of a woman except in cases of emergency" (1997b: 29). Definition of emergency in childbirth is a very controversial issue and this blanket use of "emergency" would appear to deem the woman voiceless. These statements raise very pertinent issues regarding power and control.

One of the most interesting policy developments in Irish maternity policy since the Mother and Child Scheme over 50 years ago is in relation to the situation which has been developing in the North Eastern Health Board since 2001. At the end of February 2001, the NEHB was forced to suspend maternity services at Monaghan General Hospital and Louth County Hospital due to the withdrawal of insurance cover by the Irish Public Bodies Mutual Insurance. There was much controversy, media attention and political lobbying in the wake of those closures. In May 2001, the Maternity Services Review Group was established under the Chairmanship of Patrick Kinder following the rejection of the first review of Maternity Services by the North Eastern Health Board (the Condon Report). The Kinder Report is a very important document as it provides a blueprint for a woman-centred, quality maternity service, which is safe, accessible and sustainable. It is revolutionary in the Irish context as it is concerned with empowering women, both mothers and midwives. In summary, the report recommends:

- That maternity services in the NEHB be organised on a regional level. In practice, this means that Our Lady of Lourdes Hospital in Drogheda would become a Level 3 obstetric unit which would be on a par with the three major Dublin maternity hospitals in terms of provision of services.

- A Level 2 obstetric unit would be based in Cavan General Hospital which would provide the services of a Level 3 hospital with the following exceptions: no long-term intensive care; women with complicated pregnancies, e.g. insulin dependent diabetes, would be transferred to a Level 3 hospital; and women expected to deliver before 32 weeks with an estimated fetal weight of 1,500 grams or less would be transferred to a Level 3 obstetric hospital.

- The revolutionary aspect of the Kinder recommendations is in relation to the establishment of midwife-led units in both Cavan and Drogheda, with the phased opening of units in Dundalk and Monaghan as soon as possible. This would involve the provision of ante-natal, intra-partum and post-natal care to women defined as low risk, and provision of midwifery services in the community which will provide a home birth team linked to the midwifery units.

- An inter-hospital transport service with the capacity to deal with emergencies.

- The establishment of a region-wide consumer committee for maternity and childcare services. This would enable consumer organisations to be involved in consultation about present operations and future developments and should be able to assess the quality of the services being provided.

- That organisational arrangements must provide for multi-disciplinary clinical audit.

Following the acceptance of the report in its entirety by the NEHB, a task force was established to formulate an implementation strategy for the Kinder Review Group's recommendations and to oversee their implementation. A particular concern is the establishment of regional consumer committees. In the wake of the many controversies in the health services in the NEHB, this is a crucial development.

Hospitalisation and Mortality: The Debate

Many accounts have been written of how birthing patterns and policies have changed over the past two decades. O'Connor (1992, 1995) and Kennedy (1998) in Ireland, and Oakley (1980), Wagner (1994) and Tew (1995) among others elsewhere, have recorded how women have become disempowered as the medical profession has taken over and marginalised both midwives and the informal community supports. Debate on the safety of home births as compared with hospital births has raged across continents. It is commonly argued that maternal and perinatal mortality have declined in line with the decline in domiciliary birth and the increased hospitalisation of childbirth. However, Tew (1995) and others have documented that there is not the direct cause and effect relationship which is usually presented. Looking at studies undertaken internationally for countries as diverse as the United States, Holland and New Zealand, and for births in the United Kingdom historically, Tew raises doubts about the taken-for-granted safety of hospital births. Factors which have led to a decline in the maternal mortality rate include nutrition, healthier women, bone structure, environmental factors, hygiene, education and pharmacology. Tew demonstrates that in Britain, a decline in maternal mortality was linked to different factors in different eras. In the nineteenth and the early twentieth centuries, the main cause of maternal death was puerperal sepsis. Evidence for Ireland shows that the decline in sepsis was linked to the introduction of such disinfectants as Dettol. In Ireland, the spread of sepsis was associated with medical students and nurses not washing their hands and thus carrying the disease from woman to woman (Murphy-Lawless, 1998a). Tew (1995: 92) indicates that the major cause of the decline in maternal mortality in the 1930s was the advancement of pharmacology and in particular the introduction of the drug Prontosil, which was an antibiotic used for ailments including urinary tract infections. Tew points to another reason for the reduction in the cause of maternal death as being linked to the reduction in the incidence of toxaemia. Another important development was that the detection and treatment of anaemia became possible during the 1940s. As demonstrated in Chapter Three, 75 per cent of mothers giving birth in the Coombe in 1950 were anaemic (Feeney, 1950).

Tew questions the correlation between place of birth and mortality patterns for mothers and neonates. There are other risk factors besides place that must be considered as variables. These include higher parity, socio-economic group and age group. Mortality rate according to place of birth can only be clarified if weighted according to risk factors. The factors described only begin to have meaning when they can be related to each other (Tew, 1995: 252).

> If the effectiveness of alternative services or alternative treatments is to be compared, the groups of births receiving them should have comparable risk status . . . if the outcome for these mothers is to be compared with that of another group having an alternative treatment, their combined predicted risk status from all known factors must be similar for the two groups (Tew, 1995: 256).

Retrospective Studies

The results of the 1970 Births Survey in Britain were analysed by Tew using the risk scores used by the survey's researchers. Tew showed that, except for women at the very highest risk, birth was safer at home, or in a general practitioner unit, than in a hospital (1995: 265):

> When an association exists between two conditions there is always a temptation to assume that one condition is the cause of the other . . . correlations between time series in which there is a trend in each of the related variables (and this is the case in most time series) are more likely than not to be spurious (1995: 267).

As maternal deaths have declined, mortality issues are now mostly concerned with perinatal deaths. There is concern with morbidity rather than mortality. Campbell and MacFarlane (1995), in *Where to be Born? The Debate and the Evidence,* review the findings regarding risk and benefits of giving birth in different settings using manual searches, Mediline, and the Bath University Interactive Data Services (BIDS). The first edition of their work (1987) is described by the House of Commons Health Committee report on maternity services as "the most recent and convincing work in this area, and work which has, as far as we are aware, not been substantially challenged". Campbell and MacFarlane (1995: 31) indicate how parents' views regarding care are also considered as indicators of successful birth outcome. They point out that perinatal mortality is concerned with congenital abnormalities incompatible with life and pathology associated with low birth weight. They indicate that the dichotomous debate between home and hospital births is erroneous:

> There are also considerable differences between the staff within each profession in terms of their clinical skills and experience, their ability to work with others and their skills in communicating with parents. This may well be the crucial factor rather than the setting in which birth takes place (1995: 32).

Campbell and MacFarlane argue that the number of home births is so low that it is not possible to do a randomised controlled trial. After a critical appraisal of the evidence to date, they indicate that "there is no evidence to support the claim that the safest policy is for all women to give birth in hospital" (1995: 119). The decline in perinatal mortality cannot be explained wholly or partly by a cause-and-effect relationship with the increase in hospital deliveries. Due to lack of data, it is not possible to confidently make assertions on the risk of death to low-risk women in different settings. There is evidence to suggest that morbidity is higher among women and babies cared for in an institutional setting, and there is a possibility that for some women the iatrogenic risk associated with institutional delivery may be greater than any benefit involved (Campbell and MacFarlane, 1995: 119).

Tew (1995) analysed statistics for birth in the Netherlands according to place of birth. In the Netherlands, around 30 per cent of births take place in the women's own home where a midwife or general practitioner can care for them. In hospital, midwives or obstetricians can care for them. Looking at perinatal mortality in terms of place of birth and birth attendant, evidence indicates that care given by a midwife at home is safer than care by a midwife at hospital. For first-time mothers, birth at home with a midwife was the safest option.

In a 1990 study by Professor Tricia Murphy Black, Professor of Midwifery at the University of Stirling, results showed that women who have home births have fewer complications in labour, need fewer drugs for pain relief, are less likely to suffer damage to the perineum and have an episiotomy rate only a quarter of that of a matched hospital group. In Britain, the Ministry for Health in its *Changing Childbirth* Report of 1993 stated that there is no evidence to show that it is unsafe for women to give birth in their own homes and since then policy in Britain has moved in this direction. Symonds and Hunt (1996) state:

> *Changing Childbirth* is the clearest and most positive document
> and its aims are being supported by substantial funds from the
> Department of Health. . . . There is no doubt that without ex-

actly recommending a move to home birth, the emphasis has shifted firmly towards the woman's right to choose (1997: 209).

During ante-natal care a woman is designated a risk status based on age, parity, obstetric history and general medical health. How a woman is classified is based on previous caesarean section, hypertension/toxaemia, antepartum haemorrhage, duration of pregnancy, duration of first stage of labour, fetal distress (measured by heart rate and/or the presence of meconium) and breech presentation. Despite the increased medical interventions, there is no major change in the maternal mortality rates in the last 30 years in the three major maternity hospitals in Dublin (see Table 4.14). The Department of Health report *Developing a Policy on Women's Health* claims that "the maternity services in this country are of a high standard with regard to protecting the lives and health of mothers and new born infants" (1995: 34). The vast majority of births take place in maternity hospitals and this pattern has been developing over the past three decades (Table 4.11). The size of maternity units has increased (Table 4.12) along with an increased medicalisation of childbirth. This has major implications for women in terms of choice and control by the medical profession. This colonisation of the birth process paradoxically coincided with the centrality of reproduction to people's lives. As Chodorow (1978) indicates, as women have fewer children, they tend to attach greater importance to the unique experience of childbirth. In Chapter Four, evidence was presented which documents the increasing use of interventions in the birth process (Tables 4.15–4.18).

Traditionally, interventions included enemas and shaving. Since the 1970s, interventions during labour are more likely to also include artificial rupture of the membranes (ARM), infusion of Oxytocin, episiotomies, the use of pethidine, epidurals, assisted vaginal delivery using forceps and vacuum extraction and, finally, caesarean sections. All of these procedures require a woman to lie in the lithotomy position (on one's back) and both the woman and the baby need constant electronic monitoring. Clinical reports for the three Dublin maternity units examined herein show that all of these procedures are on the increase and that this pattern has developed since the 1970s. Some of these procedures are explored below.

PAIN RELIEF

Pain is something which is associated with childbirth and is expected, anticipated and feared by women. There are many types of pain relief available to the labouring woman, some of which are associated with the social model of childbirth and others associated with the medical model of childbirth. Natural remedies include massage, aromatherapy, movement, acupuncture, acupressure, controlled breathing, meditation and birthing pools. Medical remedies include air and gas, transcutaneous electrical nerve stimulation (TENS), as well as pharmacological remedies such as pethidine and anaesthesia (Simkin, 1989).

Epidurals

An epidural is a localised anaesthetic which is injected into the epidural space between two lumbar vertebrae in the lower spine. It is designed to block pain impulses and to numb the area from the waist and the lower body. Tew (1995) writes of the growth in the use of epidural anaesthesia since the 1970s. Clinical reports from the three major maternity hospitals in Dublin highlight this trend in Ireland also. Looking at the three Dublin maternity hospitals in 2000, approximately half of the births, 51.4 per cent and 48.6 per cent in the Coombe and the National Maternity Hospital respectively and 52.5 per cent in the Rotunda, were to women who were locally anaesthetised and therefore could not feel the birth of their babies (Table 4.18).

Marie O'Connor indicates how women have come to believe they need an epidural:

> These days, the biggest decision facing many pregnant women is whether or not to opt for an epidural in labour . . . we need to ask ourselves what is the problem for which an anaesthetic

in labour is the solution. . . . Anaesthetic drugs offer a pain-free labour. And women, because they fear birth, because they anticipate pain, because they feel they cannot cope, have bought into this promise. Birth by epidural is one response to the way obstetricians manage birth in hospital (1995: 4).

O'Driscoll et al. (1993) write of the direct and the indirect effects of the epidural during labour. They write that the main danger with the epidural is that:

> . . . accidental entry of the anaesthetic agent into the cerebro-spinal fluid which can lead to profound depression of the vital centres, collapse of circulation and even death. There is also the possibility of permanent damage among survivors (O'Driscoll et al., 1993: 86).

They state that the indirect consequences can include loss of mobility as well as the fact that "intractable headache following dural tap, and retention of urine requiring repeated catheterisation, are unpleasant consequences encountered more frequently than is generally appreciated in post-natal wards" (1993: 97).

There is a relationship between back pain and epidural, and other possible effects include long-term back pain, incontinence, headaches, aches and pains, and piles (Enkin et al., 2000). Caesarean sections may sometimes result indirectly from epidurals for several reasons. There is a chance that abnormalities of the fetal heart rate as a result of the epidural can lead to emergency caesarean sections:

> If an epidural is given to a woman who is not in labour, the result is that after much confusion, a caesarean section is eventually performed on a woman who is not in labour, because it is well nigh impossible to withdraw the anaesthetic before delivery . . . the effect of this is to transfer the onus to the recipient (O'Driscoll, 1993: 87).

Epidurals, if given too late, can lead to an increase in forceps deliveries. Tew refers to evidence that epidurals can lead to prolonged labour:

Because impaired function of the uterine muscles obstructs the natural rotation and descent of the fetus and prevents the mother's urge to push, labour is prolonged and the need for forceps assistance, with its attendant dangers to the child, is greatly increased (1995: 174).

Marie O'Connor asks, "have obstetricians themselves created the need for epidurals?" and claims that "the relief of pain is also the control of labour" (O'Connor, 1995: 284). She states:

The relationship between pain, anxiety and control: the less the control, the greater the pain. The pain of humiliation for example, sexual or otherwise, is not widely acknowledged in obstetrics, nor is the possibility that fear could form part of what is generally regarded as "pain" in childbirth often addressed (O'Connor, 1995: 284).

Tew writes of the advantages for medical staff of dealing with an anaesthetised woman, who is conscious, without pain, "a compliant undistressed and undistressing patient" (1995: 174).

The fetus also is vulnerable to the effects of the epidural. The drug crosses the placenta and enters the baby within minutes, causing a depressing effect. Reducing the blood supply to and from the uterus can lead to fetal distress. Enkin et al. (2000) claim that virtually no data from randomised controlled trials are available to explore the possible effects of epidural on mothers or babies long term. They refer to a number of complications which have been reported as dural puncture, hypotension with associated nausea and vomiting, localised short-term backache, shivering, prolonged labour, and increased use of operative delivery and caesarean section. These they refer to as "well established complications". They refer to rare complications as including neurological sequelae, toxic drug reactions, respiratory insufficiency and maternal death (2000: 324). Possible, but as yet unproved, complications they refer to include bladder dysfunction, chronic headache, long-term backache, tingling and numbness and "sensory confusion" (2000: 324). They conclude that epidural analgesia:

... is likely to provide more effective pain-relief during labour than alternative methods, but may result in a substantial increase in operative delivery. We need better designed trials of epidural analgesia, which examine important questions about short-term and long-term effects on the mother and baby (2000: 329).

THE CUT

O'Connor (1996, personal communication) interestingly notes that there is no word for "episiotomy" in the Irish language. Women refer to *an ghearr*, or the cut. Before looking at the statistics on specific interventions, it is important to discuss the practice of episiotomy in Irish maternity units. Sheila Kitzinger describes the practice as the western equivalent of genital mutilation (personal communication, 1996). It is argued by those advocating the social model of childbirth that episiotomies are used to accelerate the birthing process and that what women in labour most need is time. In modern delivery units, time can be a scarce commodity. Enkin et al. indicate that "although episiotomy has become one of the most commonly performed surgical procedures in the world, it was introduced without any strong evidence of its effectiveness" (2000: 296). They conclude that "episiotomy should be used only to relieve fetal or maternal distress, or to achieve adequate progress when it is the perineum which is responsible for the lack of progress" (2000: 298).

CAESAREAN SECTION

While episiotomies are one type of surgical intervention on the increase in Irish maternity units, an even more extreme surgical intervention is the increase in caesarean sections (Tables 4.15 and 4.16).

A caesarean section is an operation by which a potentially viable fetus is delivered through an incision in the abdominal wall and uterus (Chamberlain, 1995: 298).

Chamberlain et al. indicate there is usually more than one indication for the necessity of a caesarean section:

> In most cases the indications are relative and caesarean section
> is carried out when it is thought that the balance of maternal
> and fetal indications will be reduced by caesarean rather than
> vaginal delivery (1995: 298).

Indications in which there is no choice include placenta praevia
and gross disproportion. Other indications include fetal distress,
severe hypertension, diabetes mellitus, haemolytic disease and
prolapse of the cord (Chamberlain et al., 1995: 298). There has
been a major shift in all three hospitals towards caesarean birth.
Although rates for primagravidae are generally higher, the figures
presented in Table 4.16 are total figures for primagravidae and
multigravidae. The figures presented in this book (Table 4.15) indicate that nationally 20.6 per cent of births in 1999 (latest available data) were by caesarean section. Enkin et al. indicate that
obstetricians differ in the extent to which they use this method
during childbirth. They argue that in addition to obstetricians operating in different societies and with different guidelines, other
factors are also relevant:

> . . . socio-economic status of the woman, the influence of mal-
> practice litigation, women's expectations, financial considera-
> tions, and convenience for both obstetrician and the woman
> may sometimes be more important than obstetrical factors in
> determining the decision to operate (2000: 404).

Chamberlain et al. argue that maternal mortality is four times
greater following caesarean sections than vaginal delivery. This is
linked to four main factors: firstly, the indication for the caesarean
section; secondly, the woman's health before and during labour,
whether or not there had been previous attempts at delivery;
thirdly, the length of labour; and fourthly, the skill of the surgeon
and anaesthetist (1995: 302). There is also an increased risk of
pulmonary embolism. This is more likely after caesarean section
than vaginal delivery. Also present are the risks of infection and

anaesthetic complications. Remote risks include rupture of the scar and intestinal obstructions from adhesions.

Complications for the fetus include the anaesthetic crossing the placenta which may depress the respiration of the infant. There is a risk of wrongly estimating the duration of gestation in which case the child could be born prematurely. There is also a risk of causing intracranial damage (Chamberlain, 1995: 303). Enkin et al. indicate that large series of caesarean sections have been reported with no associated maternal mortality. However, they warn:

> One should not be lulled into a false sense of security by this; no operation is without risks. The risk of a mother dying with caesarean section is small but is still considerably higher than with vaginal birth (2000: 362).

Enkin et al. classify the risks associated with caesarean section as risks of anaesthesia, operative injury, infection, postpartum pain, effects on subsequent fertility and psychological morbidity (2000: 362). The risks to the fetus they classify as ones associated with respiratory distress, linked to prematurity or the caesarean section itself due to miscalculation of gestational age (2000: 362).

COST

In examining developments in Irish maternity policies, and patterns of childbirth practices in maternity units, what emerges is a change in focus from home-centred, community-based midwife-led, low technology care, to a hospital-based, highly technical type of care, led by mostly male obstetricians. What has the associated cost been? There has been the increased financial cost of these numerous technical interventions, but there has also been the cost to the woman in personal terms through a loss of autonomy, respect and dignity. Women, to their cost, have learned that they need to be educated to give birth and that this education takes a very definite curriculum direction. There has also been a cost to women as midwives, as their profession has been gradually eroded and diminished in stature.

CONCLUSION

This and the previous chapter have traced the natural progression of the stages of pregnancy from conception through pregnancy and delivery, that is, through the maternity period, following the themes of ante-natal care and education, labour and delivery in an attempt to arrive at an understanding of the extent to which Irish maternity policies are woman-centred. What has emerged is a picture of maternity policies developing which have stressed the medical model as opposed to the social model of childbirth. A pattern has emerged where policies have been largely influenced by the obstetric professions and the increased availability of new technology. There has been a steady decline in the numbers of domiciliary births, and this has been an intentional policy.

The research presented since the 1970s, which indicates that domiciliary births are a safe option, has consistently been ignored. At the same time, women's demands for choice and control have been ignored. As the birth machine has rolled on and developed, Irish women are being subjected to highly medicalised interventions, including surgery, which can have very serious side effects and after-effects for both mother and baby. Childbirth has been taken from the hands of women, as mothers and as midwives, and become subject to active male management. Active labour has been replaced with the active management of labour and this has been rubber-stamped by the Department of Health in a succession of policy documents. There are large questions as to the extent to which woman is the focus of care and childbirth, which would seem to have become technology- and hospital-centered rather than woman-centred.

Chapter Seven

POST-NATAL CARE

The mother has given birth. There are now two people, mother and infant to the health professionals, mother and neonate, or two potential patients. This separation is vital for social policies as, at this juncture, maternity policies diverge from neonatal policies. The focus of this book is on the mother; therefore it is to maternity policies in the post-natal period that attention now turns. In the postpartum period, or the puerperium, which refers to the six weeks after delivery, the new mother has many needs — social, emotional, psychological, medical and physical. A useful tool of analysis for understanding how these needs are met in a fragmented way is to apply a welfare pluralist model (Johnson, 1987; Fanning, 1999) to the provision of services available to mothers. Looking at services in terms of statutory, private, informal and voluntary suggests that women are required to avail of services and support from a multiplicity of sources. This leads to an analysis of Irish women's experience post-childbirth, as new mothers in the context of health policies and the social supports available to them. The concepts presented in previous chapters — language, time, fear, fragmentation, choice, control, dignity, cost, power, place, health and safety — are employed in this analysis. The chapter argues that what exists in Ireland is a medical, as opposed to a social, model of care for women in the post-natal period.

FRAGMENTATION, LANGUAGE AND RESPECT

> Treating the new mother as a responsible adult by giving her
> accurate and consistent information, letting her make her own
> decisions, and supporting her in those decisions is the essence
> of effective postpartum care (Enkin, 2000: 437).

Fragmentation can involve separation, but the other aspect, the
corollary of separation, is bonding and attachment, both central to
the debate regarding the experiences of women in the immediate
post-natal period. Wesson refers to how the postpartum period
can be an immediate shock for the mother:

> For months, you and the baby have been one large, perhaps
> uncomfortable, but self-contained unit and then quite sud-
> denly you are separate. You and the baby are likely to feel the
> difference — you seem to be leaking from every orifice, you
> will be sweating a lot, starting to leak milk, weeping copi-
> ously, and surprisingly, after nine or so bleed-free months,
> bleeding heavily (1995a: 152).

Mother and baby are separate, physically. Chamberlain (1995),
like other obstetricians, views the postpartum mother as something to be managed. Wagner (1995) refers to the need for respect.
The social model of childbirth emphasises the importance of viewing woman as a complete entity, with interlinked and interde-
pendent physical, social, emotional and psychological needs. It
also tends to view the woman and her baby as a complete package and the welfare of both as mutually dependent. Wagner, referring to the complex physiological processes which take place
following childbirth, indicates that "respect for the biological
mechanisms operating in the woman and baby during the first
month after birth needs to be accompanied by an appreciation of
the social mechanisms" (1995: 210). He recounts how in the post-
Second World War period, as maternal mortality rates began to
drop, the emphasis switched to perinatal care, to the neglect of the
mother. A new role developed for health professionals, which was
to educate mothers in baby care. He claims that the hospitalisation
of childbirth gave health professionals the opportunity to scruti-

nise the infant, which he claims "gradually resulted in finding more pathology" (1995: 213).

The medical and the social models of childbirth have very different implications for women in the post-natal period. The medical model very much emphasises the mother's status as a patient and analyses her needs in terms of the physiological. Chamberlain (1995) outlines some specific areas requiring attention in the management of the mother during the puerperium as: the prevention of infection, the time of getting up, temperature and pulse, the onset of lactation, the involution of the uterus, retention of urine, incontinence of urine, cystitis and pyelonephritis, constipation, the lochia, sleep and avoidance of anxiety, diet, perineal stitches, care of the breasts, post-natal exercises, post-natal examination and family planning advice. While these areas do undoubtedly need attention and monitoring, there are other issues to be addressed. Enkin et al. (2000) refer to the post-natal period as a period in which the new mother needs both emotional support and practical help. They recognise that the form of this help is determined both culturally and historically (see Kitzinger, 1978; Kennedy and Murphy-Lawless, 2002). They point to how the increased hospitalisation of childbirth has influenced the pattern of mother–infant interaction in two ways. First of all, they point to the effects on women of giving birth in unfamiliar surroundings and who "attended by unfamiliar caregivers whom they do not know may behave differently toward their newborn child than they would at home among familiar faces" (1995: 340). Secondly, they indicate that institutional rules and policies "may obstruct spontaneous social interaction between newly delivered mothers and their babies" (1995: 340).

ATTACHMENT/BONDING

While this book is concerned with the mother, it acknowledges that attachment is a relationship of which the mother is a part. At the end of a long pregnancy, nine months of anticipation and expectation, culminating in an arduous labour, most women will want to bond, to develop an attachment with their infants (for the debate on mothers who do not feel such attachment, see Robson and Kumar, 1980; Jackson, 1994). Howe (1995), writing on attachment theory, reviews some of the literature on mother–infant bonding. Referring to Bowlby's decades of work on attachment theory, Howe argues that "whatever the weaknesses in Bowlby's early conclusions, his work has stimulated a vast amount of research and reflection on the psychological significance of the mother–child relationship in particular and social relationships in general" (1995: 49). Howe, explaining attachment in terms of nature, nurture and nature and nurture together, defines attachment as follows:

> Along with the seeking of food, fear and wariness, sociability and the exploration of new experiences (attachment) is one of a number of genetically-based behaviours designed to engage the infant with the social and physical world whilst at the same time ensuring his or her own safety. Attachment behaviour is triggered not by internal physiological needs, but by external threats and dangers. Attachment's prime biological function is to ensure that the vulnerable infant seeks protection when it feels anxious (1995: 53).

Reviewing the literature on early mother–infant contact, Enkin et al. (2000) surmise that maternal affection behaviour was more evident among mothers who had been encouraged to have liberal contact. However, they also acknowledge that where separation in the early stages does occur, its effects can be overcome in the longer term. They indicate that the restriction of early mother–infant contact can lead to breastfeeding difficulties and conclude that "most of the restrictive practices still perpetuated in some hospitals are ineffective and possibly harmful. Unless or until new evidence appears to the contrary, mothers should have unrestricted access to their babies" (2000: 437).

Enkin et al. indicate that the hospital setting, with its protocols and policies more suited to those suffering from ill health, "is not conducive either to helping the new mother develop the skills and self-confidence that she needs to care for herself and her new baby or to enhancing her sense of personal worth and self-esteem" (2000: 437). Ainsworth remarks that "despite recent research into mother–infant bonding we still know remarkably little about the processes involved in the formation and maintenance of the bond, or even the criteria that marks its establishment" (1991: 40). Klaus and Kennell (1982) highlight the pleasure experienced by a mother who has had the opportunity to hold her baby immediately after delivery. They argue that there is a critical period after birth which facilitates optimum bonding between mother and child. Ainsworth claims that such studies have led "to a revolution in obstetric ward practices that was perhaps long overdue" (1995: 39). Looking at the situation in the three Dublin maternity units under scrutiny in this book, their stated policies are shown in Table 7.1.

Table 7.1:Post-natal Practice in the Coombe, the National Maternity and the Rotunda Hospitals, 1995

The Coombe Women's Hospital

Mother and baby return to the ward together, "if mother is exhausted, she may request the baby is admitted to nursery facility to sleep". Rooming in is encouraged.

Primary nurse is assigned to each mother. Breastfed babies are brought to mother at night, if wished, though rooming in is encouraged. Glucose is banned in the hospital.

The National Maternity Hospital (Holles Street)

Mother and baby stay together unless mothers wish otherwise. Rooming in is encouraged. Primary nursing is standard. There are specialist breastfeeding staff, and lactation consultants.

Breastfed babies are brought to the mother at night if wished. Breastfed babies are not given glucose/supplements without prior consultation with the mother.

The Rotunda

Mother and baby return to the ward together. Breastfed babies are brought to the mother during the night, if wished. Breastfed babies are sometimes given glucose/supplements.

Source: Compiled by author from *A Consumer's Guide to Maternity Units in Ireland*, Irish Association for Improvements in Maternity Services (1995), second edition.

However, this does not give a clear picture as to the quality and true state of procedures, practices and the experiences of the new mother. It is important to note that one crucial variable is the availability of staff. Women have related their experiences of not being able to get out of bed to get their infants (because of stitches and other ailments) and that no staff were available to bring the infants to them. Others related their experiences of their infants being fed formula milk against their wishes, while they were asleep, and a lack of support in relation to breastfeeding (*Mother and Child 2000 Conference*, Dublin, October 1996 and the *Changing Childbirth Now* workshop, Centre for Women's Studies Summer School, Trinity College Dublin, July 1997).

TIME, HEALTH AND SAFETY

In Ireland, statutory provision of maternity care to the new mother tends to reflect the medical model of childbirth. Under the Maternity and Infant Care Scheme, a woman and her new baby are entitled to free medical care for only six weeks following childbirth and only for pregnancy-related illnesses. The mother is allocated this short time in which to recover. The *Report of the Maternity and Infant Care Scheme Review Group* (1994) recommends that a post-natal check of the mother should be carried out at six weeks after delivery by the woman's general practitioner. This, they suggest, will give the general practitioner the opportunity to offer advice to the mother in relation to family planning. It acknowledges that submissions to the Review Group advocate that cervical screening should be part of the revised scheme.

The Maternity and Infant Care Scheme allows for free medical care for mother and infant up to and including six weeks after the birth. If complications arise after this time, the three Dublin maternity units provide an "emergency" service, which they agree is totally inadequate, emphasising that there should be more community-based provision (personal communication, June 2002). Those who are entitled to medical card services can attend their general practitioners free of charge. In 2000, 30.32 per cent of the population was eligible under the General Medical Services (GMS) for medical cards. However, in 2001 only 15.6 per cent of women in the 16–44 age group were eligible (GMS, 2001). This has implications for post-natal care. It means that the remaining 84.4 per cent in this age group must depend on their own resources. A married or cohabiting woman's entitlement to a medical card is linked to the financial status of her partner. Such women who are not in paid employment must depend on their male partner for financial assistance to attend for health services. Furthermore, ineligible women who are low-paid assessed in their own right may not be able to afford the cost of €30–€50 per visit plus any prescribed medicines. This is a serious problem as it ignores the vast amount of medical research that indicates that many women suffer from pregnancy-related health problems in excess of six weeks after delivery (Blomquist and Soderman, 1991; Glazener et al., 1995; Audit Commission, 1998). It has implications also for women who breastfeed and this is particularly significant in the light of the *National Policy on Breast-feeding* (Department of Health, 1994d), as it does not allow for the occurrence of health problems related to breastfeeding.

Recent research explores patterns of women's morbidity following childbirth. Glazener et al. (1995: 282) claim that maternal morbidity is an under-researched and neglected field:

> Traditionally the puerperium has been considered to be a time of rest and rapid return to normal function. Its management has hardly altered in the past thirty years apart from a shortening of post-natal hospital stay. Changes have been ascribed mainly to differences in antenatal and intrapartum care while maternal health has deteriorated . . . many medical and behavioural aspects of post-natal health are unrecognised and hence poorly managed.

In a random study of all women delivered in Grampian between June 1990 and May 1991, maternal morbidity was measured by the mother's response to a list of possible health problems. Only 13 per cent of mothers reported no health problems after delivery (Glazener et al., 1995). Another study, by Blomquist and Soderman (1991), record only 6 per cent reporting no health problems four months after delivery.

This ill health is generally not recognised by the professionals providing maternity services. Problems including tiredness, perineal pain, breast problems, backache, piles and constipation, tearfulness and depression, anaemia, headache, high blood pressure and urinary symptoms persisted in excess of eight weeks after delivery in 69 per cent of women and between two and eighteen months in 54 per cent of women. The cumulative effect of these various complaints must add to the debilitating effect of pregnancy and childbirth on women's health and prolong their recovery. There is an underlying need for greater vigilance on the part of the professionals caring for post-natal women and also an improvement in lay and social support (Glazener et al., 1995: 285–287).

The *Report of the Maternity and Infant Care Scheme Review Group* (1997b) pays scant attention to the needs of the mother in the post-natal period, emphasising instead the needs of the newborn. It stresses the importance of the role of the general practitioner once the baby has left hospital and stresses that a visit within two weeks would re-establish the link between the mother and the general practitioner and introduce the baby to this setting. It would enable the general practitioner to complete a database, review hospital care, screening status, growth parameters and any current difficulties in management that the mother might be experiencing. This narrow focus ignores the emotional, psychological and social needs of the mother. The *Report of the Eastern Health Board Consultative Process on Women's Health* (1996) presents the issues raised by women in the Eastern Health Board area in relation to post-natal care. Their demands include:

- Close, immediate, continuous contact between baby and parents

- No unnecessary separation of baby and mother

- Babies in special care to receive as much care as possible from their parents

- Length of stay should be flexible and decided jointly by mother and doctor

- Availability of full range of family planning services including sterilisation if required

- Support for new mothers in the community.

In the Eastern Health Board Report, the Patient Advisory Council at the Coombe Women's Hospital (comprising 12 women representing a cross-section of the community, all of whom have given birth in the hospital, who make recommendations to the Master on possible improvements in the service) stresses the importance of communication, of talking to and listening to women as well as giving them information. They indicate that mothers should be respected and uninterrupted for periods of intimacy with their new babies and that staff should be trained to pick up early signs of post-natal depression. They recommend that public health nurses need to visit first-time mothers more frequently and regularly (1996: 12). They also acknowledge the potential use of the Home Help Service and the Community Mothers Scheme. In a similar vein, the *South Eastern Health Board Consultation Report* (1996) makes recommendations regarding the need for a healthy diet following childbirth, the urgent need for a mother and baby unit for women who need inpatient care as a result of conditions related to "abnormal psychological states", and also that women should be prepared for the physical, social and emotional changes that occur after childbirth.

EMOTIONAL/PSYCHOLOGICAL SUPPORT

Post-natal care and support are very important for mothers, especially for first-time mothers who make up a growing proportion of births in Ireland, numbering 40.5 per cent of all live births in 2000, an increase of 12.2 per cent since 1971.

First childbirth has a capacity that other births do not have to brand reproduction with lasting meaning for the mother, to influence all other reproductive experiences. And it is a turning point, a transition, a life crisis — a first baby turns a woman into a mother, and mothers' lives are permanently affected by their motherhood in one way or another; the child will be a theme forever (Oakley, 1979: 24).

Kitzinger refers to the limits that may be placed on a woman's choices because of the continuous and unrelenting demands of motherhood in the early stages: "with the birth of a baby suddenly a woman finds she is fixed in one role, that of a mother, and there is little choice left, because of the infant's unremitting demands on her" (1978: 36). Kitzinger acknowledges the fact that a new mother experiences a whole range of changes to which she must adjust, including changes to her own body:

> The woman is also having to come to terms with her body, which has been changing dramatically and rapidly over a short period of time, first of all swelling and becoming heavier and inhabited by another life during pregnancy, and then giving birth with all that this entails. Subsequently she is confronted with a leaking, soft maternal body, empty of the baby, but not the body with which she was familiar before the pregnancy and which she felt as uniquely her own. This is the basis of her concern, which usually starts in pregnancy, as to when she can get back to "normal". The return to normal also concerns life patterns generally (1978: 35).

Oakley echoes these words when she argues that childbirth shares features common to other major life events and "reproduction is an archetypal example of such lifechange, carrying tremendous physical, emotional, psychological and social implications for those who engage in it" (1980: 179).

This draws our attention to the wider social and emotional needs of women in the period following childbirth. Valerie Levy (1993: 148) refers to the maternity blues as the "brief period of emotional lability affecting approximately 60 per cent of women in the first week of the puerperium". Levy, asking if maternity blues is a normal occurrence, distinguishes between this experience and the more serious conditions of post-natal depression and puerperal psychosis. Reviewing the relevant literature, Levy concludes that it would appear to be a normal condition on a worldwide scale, judging the incidence of the syndrome. Without trying to arrive at an explanation for why it is so common, it is worth quoting Levy that "the blues does indeed place the mother (and her baby) at a biological disadvantage" (1993: 148). It manifests itself in crying, anxiety, tiredness, confusion, restlessness, lack of concentration, anorexia, forgetfulness and insomnia in the three to four days following delivery.

It is interesting to note that in Irish maternity hospitals, a woman is generally discharged before or at the time she is likely to experience maternity blues, and in some instances before her breastmilk has come down. So at this difficult time, when she could benefit from support and reassurance, she is sent home with a new baby to learn the skills of parenting in a potentially unsupported situation. In contrast, new mothers in Britain are visited by a health visitor every day for ten days after childbirth; and in The Netherlands, women have the opportunity to avail of a live-in nursing assistant, with special expertise in the area of maternity care and neonatal care, who undertakes domestic tasks for up to a fortnight. In Ireland, the only assistance available to women at this time is the public health nurse who is required to call once during the ten days after childbirth. The less than one per cent of women who have planned domiciliary births and employ independent midwives generally benefit from a daily visit from the midwife for each of the ten days following delivery, and usually there will be informal contact either in person or by telephone in excess of this. This continuing support is viewed as invaluable and indeed essential by mothers (Home Birth Association Annual Conference, 1998).

While the baby blues is an issue for many women, a more serious psychological condition experienced by others is post-natal depression. Research reviewed by Ball (1994) on post-natal depression indicates that there are various factors associated with it. These include obstetric problems, often linked to dissatisfaction with the management of childbirth, poor relationship with or separation from own mother, unplanned pregnancy, marital conflict, lack of a confidante, life events in year preceding pregnancy, social class and social problems. Ball warns of the dangers inherent in using differ-

ent research instruments to measure post-natal depression and outlines those most commonly used. However, for the purpose of this
book it is adequate to accept the existence of post-natal depression
as a phenomenon and to accept the fact that there is ample evidence to indicate that causal factors include a wide range of social,
physical, emotional and environmental indicators.

At the *Mother and Child 2000 Conference,* October 1996, and the
Changing Childbirth Now workshop in 1997, many women publicly
disclosed that they continued to experience emotional pain long
after the puerperium and this they claimed was due to the mis-
management of their labour and deliveries (an issue also recognised by Pigot, 1996). A similar problem was identified in Britain
by a group of practising midwives and as a result they set up an
organisation called Birth Afterthoughts. The organisation describes itself as a service for women who have unanswered questions and unresolved feelings about their birth experiences. It was
set up by a group of seven midwives in Winchester with grant aid
from The Queens Nursing Institute Awards for Innovation. It
gives women the opportunity to talk with a midwife and to read
and discuss the medical notes on their labour. The organisers are
clear in that they are providing an information and listening service and not a counselling service. It recognises the need for
women to "de-brief" after childbirth. In this context, they see de-
briefing as "a mechanism whereby women can contact the maternity services at any time after the birth of a baby to ask for information concerning the events of the birth". They recognise the
importance of narrative or storytelling, claiming that women generally want to recount their birth experiences and that "storytelling or narrative is evident every time we are faced with having
to make sense of diverse events" (Birth Afterthoughts literature).

Looking specifically at services for women suffering from
post-natal depression, the Post-natal Distress Association of Ireland (PNDAI) was established in 1989 as a self-help group to support women suffering from post-natal depression and also to
support their families. This is a voluntary organisation. Table 7.2
outlines the services which are stated as provided by the Coombe,

the National Maternity and the Rotunda Hospitals for women who are suffering from post-natal distress.

Table 7.2: Services for Women Suffering from Post-natal Distress

The Coombe Women's Hospital

If a mother, while in hospital, is perceived as being distressed, a consultation with a Consultant Psychiatrist is organised.

There is a Support Clinic for public patients who deliver in the hospital for up to twelve months post-delivery. Those with longstanding difficulties may be referred to their local area psychiatric clinic.

There is a private clinic available once a week where patients are seen for assessment and treatment. The PNDAI runs a monthly coffee morning at the hospital

The National Maternity Hospital

There is a specialist Psychological Assessment and Treatment service for post-natal depression.

Mothers attending ante-natal classes are screened for known risk factors associated with post-natal depression and when identified are referred to the Consultant Psychiatrist for assessment and treatment. The same facility is offered to those who develop depression in the postpartum period.

Ongoing treatment is provided post-discharge at either the NMH or at the catchment area hospital, as preferred.

There are plans to develop a Mother and Baby Unit for those women who require inpatient treatment as well as plans to develop improved links with general practitioner, health visitors and support groups for mothers.

The Rotunda Hospital

There is a procedure in place which allows for referral of a mother suspected to be suffering from post-natal depression where she is offered the support of the midwife, medical social worker or doctor. A psychiatric appointment can be arranged, as can follow-up treatment.

The woman will be put in contact with the PNDAI and an early visit by the public health nurse is organised. Mother is not discharged until she feels able to cope.

PNDAI support group meets here.

Source: Pigot (1996)

The picture that seems to emerge from the descriptions of services in Table 7.2 is one of hospital-based services, for the most part medical, with the back-up of the PNDAI, which is a voluntary organisation with limited statutory support. All three hospitals refer to community services, which include public health nurses, general practitioners and community psychiatric services. Noticeably absent is any reference to the role of the family as either a source of support or as a unit that may need support in dealing with this condition.

Thus, post-natal depression in Ireland is viewed primarily as a medical problem. Research would tend to indicate that while there is a medical basis to some types of depression, it can in fact be very strongly related to social circumstances and in particular to lack of social support (Enkin et al., 2000). The PNDAI outlines a suggested post-natal depression policy, indicating that what is needed is for the statutory sector, voluntary organisations and maternity services to work together to provide greater levels of support for women sufferers and their families. The PNDAI views a mother's experience of post-natal depression in the context of her role as carer, as earner as well as lifegiver:

> The pressure to go back to work or to stay away from work are equally damaging to a mother's mental health after having a baby. We must work towards more economic and social support for mothers as they face the conflicting dilemmas which motherhood can bring . . . post-natal distress is not simply a woman's complaint. We must recognise the pain and distress that it causes to partners, families and friends. We all need greater education and a more realistic attitude to childbirth and parenting. All mothers deserve support (Pigot, 1996: 72).

FAMILY SUPPORT

Ireland is a conservative/corporatist-type of welfare regime, in which the principle of subsidiarity has historically been very important. The role of the family has been prioritised as one of caring for its constituent members and in Ireland the woman was prescribed the task of carer. In the post-natal period, who cares for the mother who is herself caring for a new infant while at the same time coming to terms with some of the physical aspects of the post-natal period? In the past, childbirth was a time when women were guaranteed support and assistance from other women in the community, from female relations in the extended family, from neighbours and from friends (Kitzinger, 1975). With the changing structure of Irish society, this assistance and support are no longer guaranteed.

McCarthy suggests that "there is no longer any such phenomenon as a singular, universal family form which characterises families in Ireland" (1995a: 7). Kiely indicates that "probably the most striking feature of the family in Ireland over the past few decades is the rapid rate at which it is changing" (1995: 11). He identifies this as part of the social change which has been occurring in Ireland since the 1960s. Figures presented in Chapter Four of this book (Table 4.9) show that in 2000, 31.8 per cent of births (17,235) were to women who were not married. Flanagan and Richardson's study of unmarried mothers who delivered at the National Maternity Hospital indicates that "the title 'unmarried mother' is invariably associated with the term 'lone parent', and evokes the image of a woman deserted by the putative father of her child" (1992: 29). They indicate that "more often than not, however, this is not the case; many unmarried mothers are involved in steady on-going relationships and many others are in, what has been termed, a paper-less marriage". Oakley (1992: 36) refers to the assumption that married mothers were supported while unmarried mothers were not. She refers to Schaefer et al. (1981) who distinguishes between emotional, tangible and informational support. Emotional support includes intimacy, attachment and reassurance. Tangible support involves direct practical help while informational support includes giving information and advice, which could lead to problem-solving.

Kiely (1995) refers to the *European Community's Observatory on National Family Policies* as referring to the family as a "person-supporting group". With reference to the new mother in Ireland,

who is doing this person-supporting? Pigot, reviewing the literature on post-natal depression, concludes that it consistently indicates that women who have a poor relationship with their partner
tend to suffer (1996: 19). Factors can vary from a father being of
little practical help in caring for the baby to problems in terms of
communication, appreciation and demonstration of affection.
Kiely, writing on fathers in families, suggests that "there is concern about the more general lack of participation of men in
household tasks and child care within the family" (1995: 147).

On a European level (Commission of the European Communities, 1993: 95), both men and women agree that dressing children,
changing babies' nappies, feeding children, taking children to the
doctor, are tasks more of a "maternal nature". On the other hand,
tasks men are more likely to perform, such as playing sport (a leisure task) and punishing children are more of a "paternal nature".
While men are inclined to view these tasks as separate, women
tend to see them as the responsibility of both parents. Tasks particularly relevant to this book are those of changing babies' nappies, dressing the children/choosing their clothes and feeding the
children. Looking at the first task, something that has to be done
about six times a day for a young baby, sometimes in the dead of
night, the Eurobarometer study found that in the EU, of people
questioned, 35 per cent believed that this was a maternal task, 0.5
per cent a paternal task while 63.4 per cent felt that it was a parental task. For Irish respondents, the figures were 43 per cent, 0.3 per
cent and 56.1 per cent respectively. For the second task, that of
dressing the children, the figures are, in the EU, 43.9 per cent as a
maternal task, 0.6 per cent a paternal task, and 54.1 per cent as a
parental task. In Ireland, the figures are 47.2 per cent, 0.7 per cent
and 51 per cent respectively. For the third task, that of feeding the
children, the EU figures are 31.1 per cent as a maternal task, 0.6
per cent as a paternal task, and 67.3 per cent as a parental task,
whereas in Ireland the figures are 35.1 per cent, 0.7 per cent and
63.6 per cent respectively. Thus, for all three tasks Irish respondents placed more responsibility on the mother than the European
average.

Kiely (1995) attempts to explain the lack of change in the sexual division of labour in the home by drawing on research carried out by Clancy and Nic Ghiolla Phadraig on mothers' perceptions of the traditional roles of husbands and wives. Looking at mothers' statements regarding fathers' involvement in childcare, what becomes apparent is that apart from household repairs, fathers did very few other household tasks. Regarding childcare, mothers carry most of the responsibility. Regarding fathers:

> Interestingly, it is the more pleasant tasks of playing with the children and going on outings with them that they score the highest. In all the other duties, especially the more difficult ones such as discipline, helping with homework, getting the children to bed and attending parents meetings in school, fall on the mothers (Kiely, 1995: 149–150).

Kiely notes that this is consistent with the findings of the European Childcare Network (1990: 1–2). In Kiely's own study, 65.2 per cent of women said that the father would become more involved if she was sick or in hospital (1995: 151). Of the 284 mothers who had worked or were presently in employment outside the home, 67.7 per cent said that their involvement in housework had not been affected by their outside work. He indicates that "it is reasonable to expect that if a mother is employed outside the home that there would be a higher rate of participation in household tasks than if she were a full-time housewife. This was not the case" (1995: 53). Interestingly, Kiely demonstrates that a mother's role within the family tends to be "a separate maternal identity" while the father's identity within the family is bound up with his role of spouse and:

> . . . a picture emerges of fathers whose identity within the family is bound up with their identity as spouse. Their parental role is an extension of their spousal role. It is parental, not paternal (1995: 156).

McCarthy refers to the fact that, despite the prevalence in the media of discourse around men's increasing involvement in sharing childcare and domestic work, most of the literature "continues to cite men's under-involvement in both" (1995b: 80), quoting a male client in therapy as saying "ours is a marriage of give and take. She does all the giving and I do all the taking". Women in the post-natal period need practical and emotional support. In the absence of social support, which may have occurred with changing family and community structures, the informal sector, voluntary groups and some private entrepreneurs would appear to have stepped into the void. Before looking more closely at such initiatives, the role of statutory support will be explored.

STATUTORY SUPPORT

In Ireland, social and medical support for the new mother when she returns home is the responsibility of the public health nurse. The Institute of Community Health Nursing (information leaflet) describes the public health nurse as one who has been a registered general nurse for three years, a registered midwife for two years, has a minimum of three years' post-graduate experience and must have completed a Diploma in Public Health Nursing. The public health nurse is based at the local health centre and is a member of a multi-disciplinary team working with a general practitioner and area medical officer, home help organiser, occupational therapist, psychiatric nurse, social worker, speech therapist, voluntary and statutory agencies, and the community welfare officer. The Institute of Community Health Nursing explains the job description of the public health nurse as follows:

> The public health nurse works in partnership with the individual, family, and the community in promoting health. She manages a range of services concerning health needs through advancing years.

Government policy on the public health nursing service is laid out in the Department of Health 1966 circular on *District Nursing Services* (27/66). The 1994 report of the National Public Health Nursing Committee, *A Service Without Walls*, indicates that "maternity aftercare has become more important as the length of stay after delivery drops and mothers go out into the community earlier" (1994: 30).

The Child Health Care Service, Mothers' Views (McCluskey et al., 1996), a research report carried out by members of the Sociology Department of UCD on behalf of the Institute of Community Health Nursing, attempts to identify how mothers of infants view the health services available to them and, in particular, how they view the work of the public health nurse. The findings, based on focus groups held in seven of the eight health board areas, conclude that mothers found the first visit from public health nurses useful and supportive at a time when the mother may be feeling isolated. There was a feeling that the public health nurse was there to assess the parents' ability to care for the infant, while others were surprised at her visit, as they did not know that the public health nurse would call or had any role in relation to the newborn infant. It was felt that the role of the public health nurse should be explained during the ante-natal period, that perhaps an introduction could be made during pregnancy and that the public health nurse should telephone the mother before she calls. There was a lack of satisfaction with both the frequency and length of visits. Mothers felt that the first visit should occur as soon as possible after discharge from hospital. At present, the public health nurse has a statutory duty to visit the mother within 48 hours of notification of birth.

Some mothers in the study expressed a feeling that public health nurses were of little use in relation to breastfeeding support. There was discontent in relation to the facilities of health clinics, standards of cleanliness, also the timing of clinics, pointing to a need for evening, Saturday and drop-in clinics alongside the provision of crèche facilities. Importantly, the majority of participants felt there was a lack of reference to the mother's health, with all of the attention focused on the infant's health. Even less attention was given to mothers who had previously given birth. To demonstrate this, they refer to the tendency of mothers to refer to the public health nurse as "the baby nurse". The research pointed to a need for more emphasis on the psychological health of the mother, with a demand for advice regarding support services and organised groups for mothers and toddlers, and baby clinics.

In addition to the focus groups, a survey was carried out in which a random sample of mothers of infant children in all Health Board regions was interviewed. The interviews focused on three main areas identified as particularly relevant from the focus groups. These were mothers' views on the role of the public health nurse in childcare, mothers' appraisals of their health centres and mothers' perceptions of the role of the public health nurse in relation to their own needs. It is worth noting that the interviews were carried out by public health nurses, which may have implications for the response given as the woman's relationship with the public health nurse would undoubtedly affect her response. Also, it is important to note that the father was deemed irrelevant in this research, inferring that the mother is the sole carer for the infant and that the father's needs in relation to new parenthood are irrelevant.

In all, 387 women were interviewed with 28 per cent of them in the Eastern Health Board region, the areas in which the three maternity units examined in this book are based. Forty-five per cent of mothers expressed a belief that the best time for public health nurses to introduce themselves to the mother was before the baby was born. Another 14 per cent indicated ante-natal classes as the best time while 8.5 per cent indicated hospital after the baby is born as the optimum place. Fifty-nine per cent of mothers indicated that the public health nurse should visit at least twice a week during the first week after the baby's birth and 37.5 per cent felt that the public health nurse should visit every day during the period. Mothers stressed the necessity of the public health nurse paying attention to the health needs of mothers, with 81 per cent of them viewing this as very important (first birth) and 13.7 per cent as important. Post-natal problems referred to included post-natal blues and the mother's general emotional state, as well as problems relating to incontinence and family planning. Other areas of women's health identified as problematic included sleep, nutrition, exercise, rest and post-natal classes.

One statutory response to the changing family structure in Ireland is a programme directed particularly at young first-time mothers in disadvantaged areas. The Community Mothers Programme was originally organised by staff of the Eastern Health Board which was established to assist first- and second-time parents with infants up to one year old or two years in special circumstances. It aims to empower the mother to develop skills and confidence to "parent well". The 1997 *Plan for Women's Health* recommended that this programme be introduced on a national scale. Johnson et al. (1993) carried out a randomised controlled trial of the Community Mothers Programme with the objective of assessing whether non-professional volunteer community mothers could deliver a child development programme to disadvantaged first-time mothers for children aged up to one year. This objective is interesting, as again it tends to emphasise the child as opposed to the mother. The researchers found that children in the intervention group were more likely to have received all of their primary immunisations, to be read to daily, to play more cognitive games and to be exposed to more nursery rhymes. They were less likely to receive cow's milk prior to 26 weeks and to have better nutrition on the whole. With reference to the mothers, the study concluded that mothers in the control group also had better diets as well as a tendency to feel less tired and miserable. They were less likely to stay indoors and had more positive feelings as well as being less likely to display negative feelings.

O'Connor (1999) indicates that traditionally the experience of motherhood has been viewed as naturally positive and as a result there is no perceived need to provide support to the mother after birth. In Limerick, the Community Mothers Programme is offered to parents within designated disadvantaged areas. It is free of charge and involves up to 13 visits. O'Connor (1999: 91) concludes that "implicit in the programme, as it has developed in Limerick, is the idea that women vary in their experience immediately after the child is born". Implicit in it also is the idea that the understanding, advice and support of an experienced mother can be helpful at this time. Also present is the belief that the baby's well-being is closely related to the well-being of the mother. O'Connor, indicating that both the providers and recipients are positive, recommends that it should be extended to all other health boards.

Conroy and McDermott in their study of the Community Mothers Scheme in the ERHA suggest that the "unique feature of the Irish programme is that it is delivered not by professional health care personnel but by experienced mothers living in the same community as the recipients of the service" (2001: 1). They outline how volunteers are guided by Family Development Nurses and provided with a resource person, someone who has the dual role of being a confidante and at the same time monitoring their work. A Programme Co-ordinator, who is also a Family Development Nurse, facilitates the nurses. The Programme Co-ordinator offers specialist support, education, and management at all stages of the process. There are now 180 volunteers visiting approximately 1,100 families in their homes annually. There are also 13 parent and toddler groups. Seventy parents from the Traveller community are visited once a month. Each volunteer supports between 5 and 15 first-time mothers and meets with the FDN once each month. All the volunteers meet together every eight weeks. This is a basic group of 10–12 volunteers. Conroy and McDermott suggest:

> The volunteer mothers are volunteering with the public services for public service. The programme is a popular form of what could be called civic action. Much as the Defence Forces Reserve — the FCA — is a voluntary form of action to support the nation, the community volunteers mothers are supporting mothers (2001: 1).

Another study of the Community Mothers' Programme (Fitzpatrick et al., 1997) explored the extension of the programme to the Travelling community in Ireland and in 2002 Kennedy and Murphy-Lawless suggested that the Programme could be adapted to meet the needs of refugee and asylum-seeking mothers. The 1997 study findings are very interesting in that they suggest that the diet of the Traveller mothers was superior to that of the settled control group, and similar to the settled intervention group. Traveller and intervention mothers were less likely to feel tired, feel miserable and want to stay indoors. These findings could be due to cultural factors rather than to the Community Mothers Programme. Another interesting finding was that Traveller mothers were less likely to introduce cow's milk before 26 weeks than were the settled control group.

VOLUNTARY INITIATIVES

In the absence of any comprehensive statutory support for mothers in Ireland, a number of voluntary organisations have emerged since the 1970s which are concerned with maternity services (Table 7.3). Some of these have the support of the new mother as a particular policy priority, for example Cuidiú, which offers breastfeeding support.

Table 7.3 Voluntary Groups Concerned with the Social Support of Mothers

Cuidiú, the Irish Childbirth Trust. Cuidiú, which means caring support, is a national voluntary organisation which offers support and education for parenthood, including antenatal education and breastfeeding counsellors. They also act as a link for mothers to breastfeeding support groups.

La Leche League is an international voluntary organisation which provides information and support to women who want to breastfeed their babies. La Leche League leaders are mothers who have breastfed their babies and are willing to support mothers who wish to do so. They hold monthly meetings which offer advice and support and also maintain lending libraries.

The Irish Association for the Improvement of Maternity Services (IAIMS) was established in Ireland in 1979 in response to women's expressions of their need for such a consumer group. It is concerned with parents making informed choices about their care as well as supporting the practitioner.

Association for the Improvement of Maternity Services (AIMS) is a campaigning volunteer pressure group which is affiliated to the British organisation of the same name and claims to be more radical than IAIMS.

Irish Sudden Infant Death Association (ISIDA) offers information, promotes research and provides a confidential support service. This is provided by trained staff and parents who have themselves experienced the loss of their child.

Irish Stillbirth and Neonatal Death Society (ISANDS) helps families who know their baby died prior to delivery or is likely to live only a short time after birth.

Miscarriage Association of Ireland offers support and information following miscarriage.

Post Natal Depression Association of Ireland (PNDAI) provides help for women and their families suffering from postnatal depression

Source: Compiled by the author from organisations' promotional literature

Looking at the focus of the voluntary organisations as outlined in Table 7.3, a concern addressed by many groups would appear to be breastfeeding support. Creyghton (1992) refers to the north-western area of Tunisia where mother's milk and its positive effects on the infant are described as *baraka*, a life-sustaining force. It is believed that "it is by breastfeeding, not by pregnancy, that the strong emotional bond between mother and child is created, a bond which is extended automatically to the child's siblings" (1992: 37). It is to breastfeeding that attention will now be turned.

BREASTFEEDING

The World Health Organisation states that it is the right of every woman to breastfeed her children and the right of every child to receive human milk. While the feminist movement has traditionally been concerned with women's rights, Carter identifies a lack of apparent concern with breastfeeding in feminist literature:

> This absence of feminist engagement with the politics of infant feeding has left virtually untouched a dominant construction of infant feeding problems as involving an irrational, if natural, woman who needs to be told again and again why breast is best (1995: 1).

Maher argues that in the 1960s and 1970s, maternity was not a feminist issue, in that "women were more concerned with freeing themselves from childbearing and rearing than with realising the potential of these roles as a female resource" (1992: 1). She argues that in the 1980s, while childbirth became more visible in both medical and women's circles, breastfeeding has not shared this visibility. Maher recognises breastfeeding as being a cultural issue:

> In most societies, there are strict controls mediated by the political and symbolic system, on women's sexuality, reproductive capacities, and the form and content of their social relationships. We need to ask in what way, if any, these controls affect the practice of breastfeeding (1992: 5).

Maher (1992), referring to women's rationality, questions why so many women choose to formula feed. Formula-feeding is an attempt by women to place some of the responsibility for parenting on men, in what she describes as a social and material environment hostile to women and children. She argues that it demands money from men rather than female bodily resources. She indicates that bottle-feeding in western societies is often seen as "allowing a somewhat covert shift in the sexual division of labour, and as involving the father in parenting, by beginning with its most gratifying aspects" (1992: 8). Maher highlights how successful breastfeeding is related to economic and social conditions. She indicates that "patriarchy means that the relationship between mother and child is defined or even controlled by the cultural emphasis or social institutionalisation accorded to relationships involving adult men in dominant positions" (1992: 23).

Mary Evans, in her Foreword to *Feminists, Breasts and Breastfeeding* (Carter, 1995), succinctly summarises some of the debates, which are central to a feminist analysis of infant feeding. She identifies that historically breastfeeding was more the norm in western societies, acknowledging that it may not have been the birth mother who was nursing, with the existence of breast milk banks and wet nurses. In Ireland, milk banks do not exist, while in the United States women are actively encouraged to donate to such banks. At the same time, wet nursing is viewed as socially unacceptable and indeed by many as a health risk to the infant (Fildes, 1988).

Evans frames the infant feeding issue in the context of a woman's right to choose, acknowledging that breastfeeding for the mother is not always feasible or possible. Evans suggests the debate is both "complex and paradoxical" in that, on the one hand, while children stand to benefit from breastfeeding, large commercial interests stand to benefit from formula feeding. Maher indicates that, with the polarisation in the debate between bottle and breast:

> . . . the discussion of infant nutrition has become remarkably and misleadingly over-simplified. Commercial baby milk, it is suggested, is a vehicle for disease and death. Breast-milk is sterile and safe (1992: 3).

It is this complex and paradoxical debate in which women become embroiled after childbirth.

Cost, Time, Choice and Place

In this book, the concept of cost has already been introduced and in this situation infant feeding is very much associated with cost, but on a variety of different levels. Looking at the financial aspect, breastmilk is a resource. Breastmilk costs little in financial terms, although a ready supply depends on the mother as far as possible having a nutritious diet and plenty of rest. The Nutrition Advisory Group in its 1995 report, *Recommendations for a Food and Nutrition Policy for Ireland*, promotes breastfeeding and recommends "that breast or bottle feeding should continue on demand until four to six months of age" (1995: 42). With reference to the postnatal period, the report states that:

> The mother's diet should contain an adequate intake of energy
> and nutrients. A realistic expectation of weight loss should be
> emphasised to the mother and a gradual increase in physical
> activity is recommended. If the mother is breastfeeding, an in-
> crease in fluid intake is recommended (1995: 48).

It acknowledges the constraints of low income, referring to the
tendency of low-income women to prioritise their families' needs
rather than their own. The National Health Strategy (2001: 163)
contains an action (number 9) which states that "measures to
promote and support breastfeeding will be strengthened". A National Breastfeeding Committee was established in 2002 and a review of national breastfeeding policy with recommendations to
the Minister is to be completed by the end of 2003. A National
Breastfeeding Co-ordinator has been appointed.

An average weekly quantity of infant formula can cost in excess of €15 per week in the first months of life, and for special die-
tary needs — for example, for children with lactose intolerance
who may benefit from soya-based formula — the cost can be more
excessive. Thus, in the context of the Department of Health and
Children's advice to mothers to nurse exclusively for four months,
there is a saving of approximately €240 to each mother. Looking at
the cost of breastfeeding to the commercial sector, what is it
worth? Approximately 50,000 Irish women give birth each year;
hence the potential annual sales in infant formula are enormous.
This is apart from the costs of bottles, sterilisers and other items,
which are made redundant when a woman nurses. Therefore,
formula feeding is a lucrative market. Adding to this, the fact that
formula-fed babies tend to have wetter nappies, and hence need
to be changed more regularly, there are other additional benefits
to be reaped by the babycare industry.

While undoubtedly the cost of formula feeding can be measured in financial terms, it is important to look at the cost of breastfeeding for today's mother in terms of her three-dimensional role
as earner, carer and lifegiver. Maher states that "the degree of
freedom with which women are able to manage breastfeeding ap-

pears to depend on the configuration of roles which they are called upon to play in any given society" (1992: 29).

La Leche in their literature warn that most mothers need six to eight weeks to establish their milk supply. They advise that "the longer you can stay at home, perhaps until your baby is eating solid foods (around six months), the easier you will find continuing to breastfeed" (La Leche League of Ireland, 1992). Cuidiú, in its literature supported by the Health Promotion Unit, describes breastmilk as "the most convenient, nutritious and best value food for your baby, [which] is not available in the shops". While it emphasises the welfare of the baby, it claims "mother's milk is magic", especially in the first few days of life, referring of course to colostrum and its properties. It recognises the importance of support in the early days and claims that breastfeeding saves time:

> With mother's milk all your time is free for you and your baby — no washing, scouring, rinsing and sterilising of bottles and rubber teats, no boiling water and measuring out formula, no waiting for a bottle to warm up while baby screams. Just sit down or cuddle up in bed . . . while your milk is exactly what baby needs — clean, safe, and always at the right temperature.

This idyllic picture ignores the real difficulties experienced by women, not only in managing their time, family and work responsibilities but the physical difficulties often experienced in the early days which include exhaustion, sore nipples, engorgement and breast milk fever (Enkin et al., 2000: 454). Cuidiú literature refers to the benefits of breastfeeding to the mother, including weight loss, claiming that women who breastfeed use up the caloric value of "two aerobic workouts a week. . . . You will also get back into shape faster . . . and on the inside as well . . . as breastfeeding helps tighten up the womb again".

Time is a very important factor in the decision to breastfeed or not to breastfeed. Assuming the mother has the time, and is allowed the time, as carer and earner to breastfeed her baby, it is rarely asked what the optimum maximum length of time for breastfeeding is. The new mother in Ireland who is in the labour market has the option to take 18 weeks' maternity leave after childbirth and an additional eight weeks without pay, depending on financial resources (this is further explored later in this book). Thus, the woman who wants to breastfeed and still participate in the labour market is for the most part denied the choice to do so. This is a loss, a cost to mothers:

> Women are engaged in a complex negotiation about the control and autonomy of their bodies. All too often, and sadly, the pressures on women are such that the infant is excluded from the mother's body. It is not, therefore, that only literal loss is involved, but equally metaphorical loss of the experience and understanding of the female body as essentially different, autonomous and empowering (Evans, 1995: *viii*).

The woman who wants to breastfeed and still participate in the wider world is often ostracised, so that there is a social and emotional cost. Women generally refer to feeling uncomfortable when breastfeeding in today's society and that it is something they must do in private (Howell et al., 1997). This is visibly reinforced by the provision of baby-feeding facilities in secluded clinical settings, for example, in shopping centres. The baby-feeding room, when available, is generally adjacent to the toilets, in a room with plain walls and a hard chair. On the other hand, the woman who chooses not to breastfeed can often be labelled as selfish and uncaring towards the infant she has carried for nine months. As Evans states, "the apparently simple and essential issue of feeding infants is part of political debates about the status and role of women and the general politicisation of the body" (1995: *vii*). She indicates that "deeply felt emotions are at stake in feeding and that the sexualisation of the breast by adults fits uneasily with infant needs and demands" (1995: *viii*). Cuidiú claims breastfeeding is a natural follow-on from pregnancy and birth, maintaining the close tie between mother and baby (Information leaflet, 1994: 4). With reference to time, Cuidiú refers to how establishing breastfeeding takes time:

> Like any other new skill, it can take up to 4/6 weeks before you
> and your baby are competent and confident at breastfeeding.
> These early weeks are also known as the "learning phase"
> (1994: 4).

Again, for Irish women in the labour market, this coincides with
preparing to return to paid employment, usually when the baby is
14 weeks old, and thus the issue of weaning the infant, expressing
milk and persuading the baby to adjust to a latex teat. While it is
possible for a woman to continue breastfeeding, having introduced regular bottle feeds, mixed feeding can affect the milk supply, as the availability of milk is related to the amount and
frequency of sucking by the infant (Kitzinger, 1978). In a 1999
study conducted on behalf of the Employment Equality Agency,
women who had returned to work reported difficulties in relation
to insufficiently long maternity leave, lack of facilities as well as
lack of support from colleagues. Only one woman reported knowing about health and safety legislation as it applied to breastfeeding mothers.

Control and Autonomy

Carter (1992) writes that concern with infant feeding is also a concern with the behaviour of women. Evans claims that:

> Of all the many instances of the body as a locus of political strug-
> gle, the debates about the breast, and breast-feeding, provide one
> of the clearest examples of the body which is part of Western,
> twentieth-century experience. Thus the female body as a site of
> adult heterosexual pleasure is divorced from the body as a
> source of infant pleasure and gratification (1995: *viii*).

Jelliffe and Jelliffe (1978: 204) identify the reasons for the decline in
breastfeeding as including urbanisation and industrialisation, an
increase in women working outside the home, changing family
structures, scientific developments, ease assumed to be associated
with bottle feeding, lack of government encouragement through
crèches, limited maternity leave and at the same time the provision

of infant formula through the health services. Other factors they identify are increasing hospital deliveries and marketing and advertising of formula. In the course of writing this book, I came into contact with public health nurses who reported receiving gifts and being taken on outings by formula milk companies. Similarly, women constantly report the availability and handiness of ready made-up bottles of infant formula in Irish maternity units.

Carter indicates that the experience of breastfeeding has rarely been looked at from the viewpoint of the mother. She claims that breastfeeding offers a major challenge to feminism in that feminism is torn between minimising gender differences and emphasising gender differences (1992: 14). Does bottle-feeding liberate the woman from her biology or make her a target for commercial interests? Jelliffe and Jelliffe claim that "as with cigarette smoking, bobbing the hair, and the contraceptive diaphragm, the feeding bottle was often visualised by the 'flapper' of the 1920s as a symbol of liberation and freedom" (1978: 189). However, Carter indicates that the post-1968 women's liberation movement was more inclined to emphasise the naturalness of breastfeeding (1995: 14). She explores the concept of space, both private and public, in terms of breastfeeding and women's bodies. She explores sexuality in breastfeeding literature. Literature on sexuality as linked to breastfeeding includes literature from sexologists, in that the breasts are erogenous zones. Other writers view breastfeeding as part of female sexuality, pleasurable and autonomous. Kitzinger (1980), writing of Ireland in the 1970s, relates a tale worth quoting here. Lamenting the fact that in Ireland in 1978 the breastfeeding rate for women was 20 per cent, she writes:

> An Irish journalist attended a chapter meeting of her union taking her baby. When he cried she tucked up her jumper and fed him. At a subsequent meeting she was criticised for doing so by male colleagues, many of them fathers of large families. A father of four exclaimed, with a guffaw, "But all the same she has the best you-know-whats this side of Bantry Bay!" and this was followed by laughter and further ribald comment (Kitzinger, 1979: 205).

Unfortunately, similar comments are common 20 years later. In the course of this research, this author encountered many women who recalled similar stories and in some cases threats of violence.

In Ireland, the *Plan for Women's Health* states that "breastfeeding is regarded as the most desirable method of infant feeding because of the way it strengthens a baby's immunity to illness and also the benefits it can bring to the mother/baby relationship" (1997a: 34). It acknowledges women's concerns, expressed during the consultation process as including a perception in society that breastfeeding is primitive; that early in pregnancy women need encouragement to consider breastfeeding; that women need help and support and should not be made feel guilty or inadequate; and that in the early stages there is a need for understanding nurses. The plan queries the practice of providing free artificial milk in maternity units and its influence on women's decisions in relation to feeding their babies. The 1997 *Plan for Women's Health* Report claims that the Health Promotion Unit has recently updated information and is continuing to do so, that a number of maternity hospitals and units have adopted breastfeeding protocols and have increased the expertise of nurses in a position to support mothers. Breastfeeding resource persons have been put in place in health boards. The report claims that there is a need to find ways of developing a more supportive environment for breastfeeding mothers. It acknowledges the role of voluntary organisations.

The 1997 *Report of the Maternity and Infant Care Scheme Review Group* refers to the National Committee to Promote Breastfeeding and claims that the review group will be fully supportive of any initiatives designed to promote and support breastfeeding. In 1992, the Minister for Health established a committee under the chairmanship of Dr Mary Hurley, Senior Area Medical Officer, Eastern Health Board, to develop a national policy to promote breastfeeding. Its objectives were to increase the percentage of mothers in all socio-economic groups who breastfeed and to increase the numbers of mothers who practise exclusive breastfeeding for at least four months and thereafter with appropriate weaning foods. It focused on the following issues: breastfeeding policy in hospitals; breastfeeding policy at community level, including the role of voluntary support groups; the training of health professionals; the promotion of the support for breastfeeding in the wider community and the setting of targets for implementation and monitoring of the policy. The Committee included members of La Leche League, Cuidiú, and professionals from hospitals and the Health Promotion Unit. While it included a member of the Council for the Status of Women, interestingly it did not include any midwives, hospital-based or domiciliary, nor did it include public health nurses from the community. In 1994, the Department of Health in Ireland launched a Breastfeeding Policy which recommended that the following targets should be reached:

1. An overall breastfeeding initiation rate of 35 per cent by 1996 and 50 per cent by the year 2000

2. A breastfeeding initiation rate of 20 per cent among lower socio-economic groups by 1996 and 30 per cent by the year 2000

3. A breastfeeding rate of 30 per cent at four months by the year 2000.

The policy document suggests that the main lead in co-ordinating and implementing the Group's recommendations should be undertaken by the Health Promotion Unit of the Department of Health. This should be done in conjunction with other relevant divisions within the community, such as the Secondary Care Division and the Community Health Division. It envisaged achieving its targets through introducing breastfeeding policies and lactation teams to all maternity units by early 1995, by having in place by early 1995 the national structures necessary for Ireland's participation in the *Baby Friendly Hospital Initiative* and by having in place an identified breastfeeding resource person in each community care area. It recommended that the Health Promotion Unit Budget plan for 1995 should include provision for the designation of the unit as a National Breastfeeding Resource Centre and that from 1995 all courses for health professionals should incorporate certain recommendations on training contained in the report. It recommended that regarding the 1996 review of the Council Directive 92/85/EEC on the introduction of measures to encourage improvements in the safety and health at work of pregnant workers, and workers who have recently given birth or are breastfeeding, Ireland should support the extension of such leave to 16 weeks, and that by the year 1997, the social and health education programme in primary and secondary schools should contain a component on breastfeeding along the lines recommended in this report. It recommended that by 1998 the public sector, and in particular the health sector, should be giving a lead in the provision of workplace crèche facilities and lactation breaks.

The Current Situation

The Health Promotion Unit of the Department of Health is responsible for breastfeeding research and promotion. I contacted the unit in June 2002 for an update on developments in the promotion of breastfeeding since the policy document in 1994. There now exists a National Committee on Breastfeeding, under the Chairmanship of Professor Miriam Wiley, ESRI, which was established in 2002. Its members include representatives from NGOs, maternity units, the Institute of Obstetrics and Gynaecology and the National Breastfeeding Co-ordinator among others. Its terms of reference are to review the 1994 National Breastfeeding Strategy and to identify recommendations not yet implemented; to identify those organisations charged with responsibility for its implementation; and to engage with such organisations to establish commitment and advise on best practice. It is to provide recommendations to the Minister for Health and Children on what further action is required at national, regional and local level to improve and sustain breastfeeding rates. It is to identify other relevant areas requiring support (e.g. research, data collection, monitoring etc.) and recommend measures for their implementation. It is to report to the Minister on its findings.

Communication with the National Breastfeeding Co-ordinator in June 2002 indicates that, so far, no Irish maternity unit has achieved the status of a Baby Friendly Hospital although there are currently 22 units registered and at various stages of the process. The latest available data indicate that in Ireland the breastfeeding rate is 36.7 per cent on discharge (1999 perinatal statistics). There are currently eight clinical midwife specialists in posts throughout the country. These are resource people with a co-ordinating role. Some of the problems identified by the National Breastfeeding Co-ordinator include that there are no statutory supports in the community and no supports to span hospital and home. There is no statutory system where experienced mothers who have breast-fed successfully can pass on their experience to other women.

The breastfeeding policy report recognises that incidence and duration of breastfeeding is related to some salient factors such as socio-economic class, standard of education and attitudes of the father. Importantly, it acknowledges the relationship between mothers returning to paid employment and the cessation of breast-feeding. It recommends longer maternity leave in light of the 1996 review of the Council Directive 92/85/EEC on the introduction of measures to encourage improvements in the safety and health at work of pregnant workers and workers who have recently given birth or are breastfeeding, and refers to the need for lactation breaks and workplace nurseries. It emphasises the need for work-place facilities for expressing milk. Expressing milk can be a diffi-cult task for some women and while a successful end result can provide a food source for the infant, it does not produce the emo-tional and psychological factors associated with breastfeeding itself:

> Breastfeeding brings the mother and infant physically close and when successful is very satisfying to both. The mother–infant relationship is facilitated by the ongoing somatosensory contact involved in breastfeeding. The mother's level of en-dorphins increases significantly during suckling, which pro-motes a sense of well-being and a feeling of relaxation (Department of Health, 1994: 24).

Rather, it reduces the role of the mother to that of a food source rather than a vital, nourishing source of love and comfort for the baby.

> Mothers should be encouraged to practice exclusive breast-feeding for at least four months and thereafter with appropriate weaning foods. . . . Mothers should be advised that there are very few medical reasons for discontinuing breastfeeding (Department of Health, 1994a: 9).

While there may be few medical reasons for discontinuing breast-feeding, there are definitely social reasons for doing so.

The Innocenti Declaration on the promotion, protection and support of breastfeeding was produced and adopted by partici-pants at the WHO/UNICEF policy-makers meeting on breastfeed-ing in the 1990s, a global initiative held in 1990. In September 1992, the Irish Government ratified the UN Convention on the Rights of the Child, Article 24 section 1:

> State Parties recognise the right of the child to the enjoyment of the highest attainable standard of health and to facilities for the treatment and rehabilitation of health. State parties shall strive to ensure that no child is deprived of his/her right to ac-cess to such health care services.

> **Article 24 Section 2(e):**
> State parties shall pursue full implementation of this right, and, in particular, shall take appropriate measures, to ensure that all segments of society, in particular parents and children, are informed, have access to education and are supported in the use of a basic knowledge of child health and nutrition, the advantages of breastfeeding, hygiene and environmental sani-tation and the prevention of accidents.

Wiley and Merriman, in their 1996 national study *Women and Health Care in Ireland*, indicate that 59 per cent of mothers never breastfeed. Almost half of the women who do breastfeed do so for less than six weeks, while a quarter breastfeed for three months. Over 12 per cent breastfeed for over six months. Almost one-quarter of mothers consider that they were made to feel embarrassed by breastfeeding, while a staggering 83 per cent agree that breastfeeding facilities in public places were inadequate. Twenty per cent of mothers aged 35 to 45 breastfed their babies, whereas in the 18–25 age group, 85 per cent of mothers have never breast-fed. Mothers with higher educational levels are more likely to breastfeed. Older mothers (35–44) breastfeed for longer. Probability of breastfeeding increases with age, education and parity. Ten per cent said more help from health visitors or nurses would have helped them to continue breastfeeding. Wiley and Merriman indicate that social class differences in the reasons for stopping breastfeeding were not significant (1996: 134). Returning to work was cited by 8.7 per cent of mothers as the reason they stopped breastfeeding. While this figure may seem low, it reflects the fact that most women do not manage to continue breastfeeding until they reach that stage for a plethora of reasons, some of which have been addressed above. The most common factor for stopping breastfeeding, cited by 21 per cent, was "baby not getting enough" which is a very important issue as a mother's breastmilk supply is directly dependent upon the mother being well-rested and well-nourished.

Howell et al. (1997), in a study of breastfeeding rates in the North Eastern Health Board region, found that, of 287 women, 34.8 per cent were breastfeeding at birth, 29.6 per cent on discharge from hospital, 20.2 per cent at six weeks and 10.1 per cent at 16 weeks. Of those who bottle-fed, 27 per cent did not want to breastfeed, and 18 per cent felt it was too time-consuming. Twenty-four per cent were unable to give any benefits for breastfeeding and 9 per cent said there were no benefits. Of those who did breastfeed, 54 per cent felt that people wanted them out of their sight, while 22 per cent stopped due to poor supply (a factor that is generally related to the mother being poorly nourished, tired or under stress). Nineteen per cent reported stopping because of tiredness and 18 per cent because the baby was unhappy. The researchers conclude that existing policies to increase breastfeeding have either failed or not been implemented, and that breastfeeding needs to become more attractive for mothers.

Private Provision

In recent years, there has emerged in Ireland a number of independent private lactation counsellors who are self-employed and feel that their service meets the needs of many women who are trying to master the art of breastfeeding. They describe themselves as:

> A health care professional whose scope of practice is focused upon providing education and management to prevent and solve breastfeeding problems and to encourage a social environment that effectively supports the breastfeeding mother and infant. . . . Primary focus is the provision of education, assistance and support to breastfeeding women and their families (literature issued by a private lactation consultant, 1996).

One private lactation consultant in the Dublin area offers a "total care package", which includes private consultation, six ante-natal classes, two home visits and introductions to a mother and baby group and unlimited attendance at a cost of €200 plus travelling expenses. It seems incredible that a woman has to pay this amount for such a basic service which is taken for granted in many other European countries, especially in the light of our National Breastfeeding Policy. Voluntary groups such as La Leche provide many of these services for free.

CONCLUSION

Women as new mothers, who may be suffering at least from exhaustion, look to a multiplicity of sources for support — social, emotional and physical. These sources reflect the social divisions of welfare, the statutory, voluntary, and informal sectors. In a society where post-natal care has been identified as the responsibility of the medical profession, i.e. obstetricians, neonatologists, and public health nurses, women again are faced with the concept of de-commodification, where those who have purchasing power can avail of the services of such independent practitioners as lactation consultants, while those suffering from post-natal depression can buy a choice of mental health services. At the other end of the spectrum, women have to depend on the public health care system and all women can turn to the voluntary sector. What becomes evident from this analysis of Irish women's experiences of the post-natal period is that, in Ireland, the medical model dominates the social model of care. However, the Community Mothers Programme is one step in the development of policies of social care. New mothers have to face many challenges associated with their new roles, with its inherent responsibilities, often with inadequate support. Such challenges include recovering from the labour and delivery, physically and emotionally; returning to the labour force; and finding affordable and adequate childcare. For some mothers there is the fear of how the infant will suffer if she herself cannot or chooses not to breastfeed. Others have to overcome the fear associated with breastfeeding, the fear of where, when and how to do it without being socially ostracised, and at the same time perhaps managing her position in the labour market. The mother in Ireland who continues to breastfeed must be a very highly motivated individual if she is to deal with the many and major obstacles that stand in her way.

Bearing these issues in mind, this book will now proceed to look at the special needs of mothers in the context of race, ethnicity, disability and lifestyle.

Chapter Eight

RACE AND ETHNICITY

This book argues that policies which affect a woman during pregnancy and the first year of motherhood should be woman–centred. While women in this period of their lives have common needs, some women have very specific and additional needs to those of the majority of service users. Drake (2001) discusses the challenges for policy formulation and implementation in a plural society with various identities, cultures and social and political sub-groups. In such a setting there are diverse values, policy principles are challenged and policy outcomes can discriminate among groups. He suggests that the challenge is to evolve principles and policies to accommodate distinct groups. Offering the same service to everyone is clearly discriminatory. Provision should be needs-led. In this and the subsequent two chapters, the maternity needs of diverse groups of women in Irish society during the maternity period are explored.

The National Economic and Social Forum (NESF) refers to "the complex interactions in the public and private spheres of people's lives" (2002: 3). This book has argued that pregnancy and the first year of motherhood is an example of where the private and public aspects of women's lives meet. The NESF report argues that significant steps have been taken in Ireland in recent years towards creating a more equal society, characterised by new legislation and actions to promote equality (2002: 3). It argues that these are "among the most advanced in Europe, and are beginning to shape up as a strategic framework for action on equality" (2002: 3). The NESF report stresses that identity must be placed at the heart of a strategic framework on equality. This involves affirmation, negotiation and accommodation of diversity (2002: 24). In Ireland in recent years, multiculturalism has become very much part of public discourse. What is under discussion is usually the increased presence of asylum-seekers and refugees, despite the fact that Ireland has its own indigenous minority which has never achieved full social rights. It is to these issues that attention is turned in this chapter.

In looking at Ireland's indigenous population and oldest ethnic minority, Travellers, it is important to focus on the maternity needs of Traveller women in the context of their wider cultural and biographical experiences of living in Ireland as part of a marginalised community. Travellers in Ireland identify themselves as a distinct community with a nomadic way of life, with their own culture and traditions and their own language, "the cant". Their kinship patterns favour marrying within their own community and at a young age. They continue to suffer deep discrimination. Crowley (1999: 249) refers to a 1997 report by the Irish National Coordinating Committee for the European Year Against Racism, which indicates that "one of the more visible forms of racism is that experienced by the Traveller community based on their distinct culture and identity which is rooted in a tradition of nomadism" (1997: 5). Crowley suggests that Travellers have been defined as deviants by the settled community and are viewed as "failed settled people in need of rehabilitation and assimilation" (1999: 244). Pavee Point in its fact sheet on women indicates that "Traveller women experience an intersection of a number of oppressions and experience both racism and sexism". Quirke (2002: 7) refers to a survey on attitudes carried out in January 2000 which indicates that:

> . . . in terms of accepting or including Travellers socially or into the community, 36 per cent of Irish people would avoid Travellers; 97 per cent would not accept Travellers as members of their family with 80 per cent saying they would not accept a Traveller as a friend; 44 per cent would not want Travellers as community members (*Citizen Traveller*, 2000).

The 2000 Department of Environment and Local Government/Local Authority count of Traveller families indicates that there were 4,898 Traveller families in that year (Department of Health and Children, 2002: 21). Of this number 1,353 live in the Eastern Region Health Authority (ERHA) region.

There are strong links between socio-economic differentials, such as access to education and accommodation, and health status. Quirke, Co-ordinator of Pavee Point's Primary Health Care Project (Pavee Point, 2002: 6), indicates that some research carried out since the latest national study on Travellers' health (conducted in 1989) indicates that "the health status of Travellers has not improved, and more alarmingly may have deteriorated". A statistic she presents which is particularly relevant to this study is the fact that the Irish Sudden Infant Death Association (ISIDA) in 1999 identified the rate of Sudden Infant Death among Travellers as 12 times that of the settled population. Quirke states that "the issues around health are inextricably linked to issues regarding appropriate accommodation provision for Travellers and further to the social and economic exclusion of this community within contemporary Irish society" (Pavee Point, 2002: 6). Accommodation is perceived as the major issue for Travellers with constant demands being made for access to suitable accommodation. Crowley (1999: 251) outlines how accommodation for Travellers to date has been characterised by inadequate provision, with one-quarter of families living on the side of the road without access to basic facilities; its unsuitability for the traditional organisation of economic activities around family and home; its inadequacy for transient Travellers; and overcrowded and under-resourced temporary sites.

HEALTH STATUS OF TRAVELLERS

Over a decade ago, the broad figures on fertility and mortality for Travellers were:

- A fertility rate of 164.2 per 1,000, compared to 70.1 per 1,000 of the settled community

- Infant mortality rate of 18.1 per 1,000 live births, compared to the national average of 7.4

- Travellers only reaching the life expectancy of that achieved by settled people in Ireland since the 1940s

- A low uptake of maternity services, with less than a third of mothers attending hospital by the end of the first half of pregnancy

- A low uptake of infant health services, immunisations and attendance at development check clinics, at less than 59 per cent

- High mobility of the Traveller community with only 50 to 60 per cent of infants located by the Public Health nurse at the child's first birthday (Barry, 1989).

Traveller women are doubly discriminated against as women and as Travellers. Therefore, it is no surprise that their health status suffers as a result. The more recent Health and Welfare of Traveller Women Baseline Study, which was completed as part of the initial Primary Health Care Project (examined further on in this chapter), indicates:

- 46 per cent of the women surveyed described their own health as "poor" or "fair".

- 34 per cent had been ill in the four months prior to the survey.

- 60 per cent had been prescribed medicine by a doctor at last once in the previous year.

- 33 per cent of the women surveyed said that they suffered from long-term depression.

- 10 per cent of the women had taken anti-depressants prescribed by their GP in the previous year.

- 32.6 per cent of the total respondents had had a cervical smear test.

- 55.1 per cent had never done breast self-examination (38.7 per cent of the general female population).

- While 69.1 per cent believed ante-natal classes were a good idea, less than 1 per cent had attended.

- 51.5 per cent of the women who had children did not attend post-natal check-ups for themselves after the birth of their last child.

- 73.4 per cent did bring the baby for a six-week check-up.

- 88 per cent had a preference for a female doctor.

- 68 per cent of women said that being able to plan the spacing of their children was very important.

- The ideal number of children was judged to be four.

- 50.3 per cent had never had family planning advice or service (data supplied by Pavee Point from unpublished Baseline Study).

As regards methods of family planning ever used, women reported as follows: the contraceptive pill, 46 per cent; intra-uterine device (IUD), 19.7 per cent; and Depo Provera, 10.2 per cent.

Examining this data, it is not surprising that health care for Travellers has been put forward by Travellers themselves as a burning issue for reform and development. However, it is only in recent years that this concern has been echoed in official policy documents, undoubtedly a result of the successful lobbying by Traveller groups and the quantifiable success of the Primary Health Care Project itself.

The National Health Strategy was published in 1994. It recognised the specific health needs of Travellers and made a commitment to supporting joint research with the *Task Force on the Travelling Community* into access to health services. The Task Force (1995) stressed that there should be specific services designed for Travellers, which would complement mainstream services and improve access to these. It also recommended the development of "peer-led services" and those primary health care services should be developed on an outreach basis. It identified the very important role of voluntary sector support groups for Travellers.

The discussion document, *Developing a Policy for Women's Health* (1995), made a specific reference to the needs of women Travellers. Recognising the importance of environmental issues in improving women's health status, it stated that improving accommodation was "a precondition for reducing premature mortality and unnecessary morbidity among Traveller women" and called for the development of services "with a special emphasis on maternal and child health". Following consultation with women at regional and local level throughout Ireland, *A Plan for Women's Health* was published. The first of its kind in Europe, this national policy for women's health recommended the development of services to address the particular needs of Traveller women.

In 1995, the Report of the Task Force on the Travelling Community recommended the establishment of a national and regional structure to facilitate Traveller participation in the health service. As a result, there is now a Traveller Health Advisory Committee (THAC) in the Department of Health and a Traveller Health Unit in each Health Board. The THAC was established at the end of 1998 and submitted proposals to the Department of Health and Children at the end of 2000. The Traveller Heath Strategy is a response to one of the recommendations of the Report of the Task Force on the Travelling Community (1995). The 2002 document indicates that up to 80 per cent of adult Travellers are unable to read. This has major implications in relation to health promotion and accessing services. The core value is to achieve equity in healthcare service provision. In this regard, it is useful to refer to the publication produced by Pavee Point, *Traveller Proofing — Within an Equality Framework*. It highlights the importance of collecting, collating and analysing data on Travellers in an attempt to improve their situation; to evaluate policies and provision and to combat discrimination (2002: 2). Ronnie Fay, the Director of Pavee Point, refers to the need for the collection of socio-economic and demographic data which can be used to help to improve the living conditions of Travellers (2002: 2).

The Primary Health Care Project for Travellers

The Primary Health Care Project for Travellers originated from Pavee Point in conjunction with the Eastern Health Board. Pavee Point is a non-governmental organisation established in 1983. It is a partnership of Travellers and non-Travellers who aim to address the needs of Travellers as a marginalised ethnic group.

The methods used by this innovative project were planned as to be acceptable to the target group and was concerned with developing culturally specific resource material, which has been very beneficial. It uses a community development approach, which has ensured that the Traveller women themselves were the most valuable component of the Project. In particular, their role as front-line workers, working with their own communities, bringing with them a wealth of sensitivity and personal experience of the complexities of life in that community. Public health nursing, environmental health and dental health were recognised as priorities for intervention (Pavee Point, 1996).

The role of the community health workers was to access and disseminate health information to the Traveller community, engage in health promotion, increase Traveller participation in health issues and to develop an advocacy role in their community. Many of its goals are directly related to health services directed at women during pregnancy and the first year of motherhood.

Training

One of the specific objectives developed was to develop the skills of Traveller women in providing community-based health services (Kennedy, 2001). The Project is also involved in in-service training to health professionals. These workshops are held at Pavee Point and also in community settings such as some of the major Dublin hospitals. The training focuses on racism, Traveller culture and health needs and such groups as ERHA dental personnel and public health nurses have attended.

The implementation report (Pavee Point: 2000) identifies the need to recognise project workers as professionals and that quality standards are identified and established. The Primary Health Care Certificate, jointly accredited by Trinity College, the Eastern Health Board and Pavee Pont, has provided the professional training necessary for the CHWs. This course incorporated the original training material and curriculum. This is the basis for the standardisation and professionalisation of the CHW role. A Trainers Training Course in Primary Health Care was developed in partnership with the ERHA, Pavee Point and the Equality Studies centre at UCD. Those who successfully complete such a course would be accepted as health professionals in their own right and would be qualified to deliver and manage a Primary Health Care Project and act as extern/peer assessor for other Primary Health Care courses. One Traveller woman completed this course in 2002.

Policy Choices and Reforms

The Primary Health Care Project has been viewed as successful in having a positive impact on take-up of services by Travellers. At the same time, it has developed an innovative model of training leading to employment of Travellers in the Primary Health Care Sector. The Implementation report concludes:

> This project has been a major success in that it presents a vision of what is possible for the next generation of Irish Travellers. The women emphasized their pride in the professional service they are providing to their own community, their satisfaction at their ability (which was validated by the certification they received from the Minister for Health) to have completed the different training modules, and imparted the information and encouragement to other Travellers. . . . They expressed the hope that their jobs will be secure so that they can get further training and develop even more skills (Pavee Point, 2000: 30).

One of the most important results of the Primary Health Care Project is its replication in other areas throughout Ireland. Projects have been set up in Limerick, Galway, Donegal and Kerry. A further possible development could involve the adaptation of this project to meet the needs of refugee and asylum-seeking women in Ireland.

The Pavee Point Fact Sheet on Health states:

> As Travellers are a distinct cultural group with different perceptions of health, disease and health care needs they require special consideration in the health service.

This is what Zweifler and Gonzalez (1998) conclude about the challenge of developing the capacity to provide accessible care to diverse and under-served populations on the basis of their expressed needs. Many of the care providers dealing with Traveller women in Ireland are acutely aware of the need to move towards these aspirations. Drawing on the wealth of experience of all of those involved in the Primary Health Care Project for Travellers is undoubtedly a good starting point. The Traveller Health Strategy (2002) proposes several important actions. The specific actions on maternity include health education programmes which will highlight the relevance of proper ante-natal and post-natal care, and the introduction of culturally sensitive ante-natal education and ante-natal care. This has begun in the Rotunda, one of the two Dublin maternity hospitals where Traveller women generally choose to give birth. The other is the Coombe. Priority will also be given to providing de-centralised ante-natal clinics throughout the country. Earlier ante-natal registration will be encouraged through the Maternity and Infant Care Scheme (shared care). Liaison between maternity units and the Designated Public Health Nurses will be improved to ensure early identification of Traveller mothers. This is to commence within six months of the publication of the Strategy. Mothers will be encouraged and supported to stay in hospital for an appropriate time post-natally. Peer-led educational and awareness programmes should be considered in relation to family planning and sexual health.

Quality Care and Diversity

In an influential review article on quality care in the human services, Paul Wilding (1994) has identified four key attributes which can be measured in the search for quality care:

- A service should be accessible to its client group

- A service should be acceptable to its client group

- A service should be effective for its client group

- A service should be open to its client group in its aims, objectives, communication and practice.

Wilding argues that quality of care is far more than practical, technical or clinical skills. Because it is ultimately bound up with how people relate to other people, quality care is far more than the sum of its parts; its provision relies on the delivery of care in the context of our human relationships. To take Wilding's analysis and apply it to midwifery care, for example, it can readily be seen that the safe care of a mother through pregnancy and birth entails far more than just her physical care and having the technical skills to confirm the course of the pregnancy and facilitate the baby's birth. The relationship between the caregiver and the woman will be the very basis of the delivery of quality care.

In the context of Traveller women, the concepts of accessibility, acceptability, effectiveness and openness take on even more meaning, for here is a group with special needs which will make special demands on existing services. It concerns the quality of the relationship the person can bring to the work which will give a woman confidence to really speak her needs and feelings. Without that dimension, it simply will not happen. The Primary Health Care Project is a step in this direction.

Many of the issues raised here are also very relevant to the many women who come to Ireland seeking asylum who are either pregnant on arrival or become pregnant while living here. It is to this group that attention is turned in the remainder of this chapter.

REFUGEE AND ASYLUM-SEEKING WOMEN AND MATERNITY CARE

In 2000, 20 per cent of births were to women asylum-seekers in the three Dublin maternity hospitals under study in this book. In the NEHB, as a result of asylum-seekers being accommodated in Mosney, ten per cent of all births to women in Our Lady of Lourdes Hospital in Drogheda in the first half of 2002 were to asylum-seeking women. The 2000 clinical report of the National Maternity Hospital indicates that the hospital provided a service to 485 people who were asylum-seekers or refugees; only 20 of these were not seen by a social worker (page 122). The Coombe records having served women from a staggering 90 countries in the year 2000. The Rotunda social work department worked directly with approximately 548 people from different ethnic groups (2000: 75). In Ireland since 1998, 6,060 non-national, non-EU applicants have been granted residency on the basis of having Irish-born children. Recently, the Commissioner of the Office of Refugee Applications has publicly stated that "between 45 per cent and 50 per cent of female asylum seekers are visibly pregnant at the time of application" (Quinlan, 2002: 1).

In 1990, an Irish court case determined that the parent of any child born in Ireland has the right to apply for the legal status of leave to remain (Fajujonu Ruling). This was strengthened in 1998 when the Good Friday Agreement confirmed the right of any child born on the island of Ireland to be granted Irish citizenship. Fuelled no doubt by much media debate and speculation in relation to women coming to Ireland seeking asylum when pregnant, the government mounted a challenge to the Fajujonu ruling of 1990. The argument was that the Fajujonus had lived in Ireland for nine years before the Supreme Court ruled in their favour as parents of an Irish-born child. Thus, a distinction would need to be made between those with a strong claim to residency, based on the time spent in Ireland, and those who have been in other EU countries before coming to Ireland and subsequently giving birth here (Haughey, 2002a; 2002b; 2000c).

Research literature on pregnancy and new motherhood presented in Chapter Two emphasises that mothers live their lives where the public and private meet at many different levels. Mothers' everyday lives are influenced by public expectations, prescribed roles, social, political, economic, and cultural constraints and circumstances while on a parallel level private, biographical, emotional, physical, and psychological experiences have to be coped with by these same mothers. Ann Oakley has argued that:

> Birth is an isolated biological episode only to hospital administrators and official statisticians; the women who give birth have a past and a future. So it is in this biographical context that childbirth has its social meaning (1979: 23).

The relevance of this biographical context for refugee women who have been dislocated from their extended families, cultures and societies cannot be emphasised strongly enough. As Muecke indicates, "refugees' lives are continuous despite major discontinuities" (1992: 519) and thus women are going on with the physical, psychological and social work of mothering despite radically changed circumstances of the experiences of being exiled. Focusing only on the time around labour and delivery is problematic, as women's lives are continuous and from the moment of conception women experience physiological changes which are part of a process which continues on through the entire pregnancy, labour, delivery, lactation and the post-natal period. For some refugee women, conception occurs as a result of rape. Others have experienced torture, and may re-experience this extreme trauma during pregnancy, birth and the post-partum period. The major life event which childbirth has become in modern societies is more complex for the woman who is fleeing persecution, who has experienced and is experiencing stress stemming from the situation in which she finds herself as a refugee.

Women who come into contact with the maternity services in Ireland as refugees or asylum-seekers will already have experienced profound loss. As Athey et al. indicate, loss is "a defining characteristic of refugee status" (1991: 7). This can vary from loss of family, community and country to problems of dealing with violence, torture and rape. This experience of loss and suffering creates special complexities for pregnant women in relation to their physiological, psychological and social needs. As Muecke indicates, their experiences prior to migration and indeed while migrating will have been "fraught with health risk and uncertainty" (1992a: 517). There is a strong possibility that experiences of health care prior to migration will have been grossly inadequate. Evidence, for example, from Bosnia indicates that from 1991 to 1995:

• Perinatal mortality rose from 15.3 per 1,000 live births to 38.6 per 1,000 live births.

• The incidence of low birth weight doubled.

• Congenital abnormalities rose from 0.37 per cent to 3 per cent.

• There was an increased percentage of neural-tube defects (Reproductive Health for Refugees Consortium, 1998).

In relation to Kosovan refugees, the Department of Health in Great Britain (1999) indicates that women there may have been without healthcare or formal assessment for some time as the formal health care system began to collapse in their homeland from 1990 onwards. Other experiences such women may have had are particularly relevant to health status. These include malnutrition, excessive stress and life-threatening situations. These can be classed as pre-migration stressors of deprivation. Athey et al. (1991: 7) argue that deprivation can include insufficient food or water, lack of medical care and suitable accommodation. Trauma, an additional stressor, can include any experiences which may be life-threatening, terrifying and/or overwhelming (Athey et al., 1991). These important issues must be viewed in the context of the experiences of women as they journey through the maternity period in a foreign country and culture and, all too often, alone.

In Ireland, the 1996 Refugee Act distinguishes between the needs of male and female refugees. References are made to persecution resulting from a person's gender or sexual orientation, and there is also recognition of sexual abuse as a form of torture. The Refugee Women's Legal Group (1998) defines sexual violence as:

> Enforced nakedness; sexually abusive taunts and threats; rape; mechanical stimulation of the erogenous zones; the insertion of objects into the body openings; the forced witnessing of sexual acts; forced masturbation by others; fellatio and oral sex; a general atmosphere of sexual aggression and threats of the loss of the ability to reproduce and/or enjoyment of sexual relations in the future.

Examples of this include reports from women who came to fear giving birth in state-run maternity hospitals because they feared forcible sterilisation. Physical health needs may include damage to the vagina and cervix as a result of rape and torture. Some of the psychological consequences may include anxiety, loss and bereavement and guilt and shame. In societies where rape has been rare, for example in Albanian communities, women will feel especially deep shame and may be rejected by their families and community members. The issues around rape and torture add even greater urgency to the development of sensitised support services during pregnancy and following childbirth (Sachs, 2000; McCarthy, 2000).

As demonstrated so far in this book, the vast majority of births take place in consultant-staffed maternity units and as the size of maternity units has increased, so too has the medicalisation of childbirth. Simultaneously, length of stay has decreased. As a result of such developments, Inch, writing in the British context, indicates that women's feelings can sometimes be disregarded in a hospital setting because "power relationships between givers and receivers of care, both in pregnancy and labour are often unequal". This, she argues, is due to the size and complexity of hospitals which are bureaucratic and hierarchically organised institutions. She argues that status and role can dominate "the more personal and spontaneous factors that characterise relationships in the less public spheres of life" (Inch, 1981: 70). This requires exploration in relation to the needs of women who are refugees and asylum seekers as they will have had a range of experiences, as well as expectations, which may be more complex and diverse than women in Ireland who will have grown up with knowledge of a specific western model of health care and maternity.

Irish Maternity Services

In the context of the large numbers of births occurring in the three Dublin maternity hospitals at present, attention has been drawn to the extra pressures placed on their limited resources by large numbers of refugee and asylum-seeking women who have very complex needs, sometimes medical but always social. Similar pressures exist in relation to support services in the community and in particular in relation to accommodation as housing shortages have become a feature of life in urban Ireland. In this context, this author with Jo Murphy-Lawless (Kennedy and Murphy-Lawless, 2002) conducted a research project in 1998–2000 on behalf of the Women's Health Unit of the Northern Area Health Board, to determine the physical, emotional and material support needs of this vulnerable group of women. This was the first substantive research carried out for women in this situation in Ireland and the United Kingdom. The objective of the research was to collect baseline data on refugee women's experiences, expressed needs and perspectives of the existing care services in order to inform the development of relevant maternity care policies for this group of women. These experiences contribute to women's care needs being so much greater than the exclusive focus on physical health in pregnancy and birth that is often implied by our model of maternity care, especially under the medical model.

The study involved 61 extended interviews with women from Nigeria, Romania, Kosova, Cameroon, Ghana, Ukraine, Algeria, Bosnia, Iraq, Poland, Russia and Sierre Leone. Language competency was varied, with West African women on the whole having excellent English. Many of the women coming from East European countries had learned what English they had on their own. The Roma women interviewed had virtually no English and here a Romanian translator was relied upon. An Albanian translator was employed for all interviews with Kosovan women. Of those women interviewed, 18 were in the latter stages of pregnancy and the remainder had already given birth. Forty-four per cent of the women were having their first baby here in Ireland. Two of these had arrived in Ireland in the late stages of their first pregnancy and were on their second pregnancy when they were interviewed for this study. A range of professional health care staff was also interviewed. Like the situation for Traveller women, maternity needs can only be addressed in the context of the much broader range of disadvantages suffered by these women.

Housing and Direct Provision

Ireland, similar to Britain, has gone over to a system of direct provision for basic material needs of asylum-seekers. Adults have a €19.05 weekly cash payment and each child €9.50 in addition to accommodation and meals. The accommodation for asylum-seekers was either hostel accommodation or bed-and-breakfast with meals or food supplied to cook each day (hostel kitchens). However, a pregnant lone woman, once she was over 32 weeks pregnancy, became entitled to basic social welfare as a prospective parent. Once her baby is born, if she is a single mother (her partner is not in the country), she can then apply for the same allowances and entitlements as Irish women in that position. This includes a basic weekly payment, plus child allowance plus a state subsidy towards rent that comprises between 50 and 70 per cent of rent levels, depending on the locality. Because of an acute shortage of rented accommodation in the Dublin area, asylum-seekers were also subject to a policy of dispersal around the country. The alternative was that very unsatisfactory initial and temporary accommodation often turned into a long-term and inappropriate housing setting.

The accommodation conditions encountered in the course of this research were absolutely unacceptable. There were usually strict conditions placed on women and families, strictest of all in hostels and bed-and-breakfast establishments. In some cases visitors were not allowed and there were strict entry times into the buildings. Single women, either pregnant or with newborn babies and small children were living either in dormitory-type conditions or sharing bedrooms. It was not possible for women to make a cup of tea in their rooms in their hostel or bed-and-breakfast accommodation. They were often hungry but were restricted to a schedule of mealtimes, which did not fit in with their pregnant and postpartum needs. The researchers never saw cots for newborn babies. The availability of cooking facilities varied often with only access to a microwave in the kitchen. Women struggled to keep their babies quiet at night for fear of disturbing others in the room.

The severe problems many women and their families encounter on a daily basis included overcrowding; for example, three women and four very young toddlers and babies sharing a room with three double beds, no cots, no toys, no storage space for personal possessions and only a tiny prefabricated bathroom space in the corner with a shower. It was not uncommon to find women and babies sharing accommodation with unknown men from a family of strangers; where some women had experienced rape, the levels of tension were palpable. The overall lack of privacy, the lack of independent living, the lack of adequate bathing facilities — no baths, only shower cubicles — the lack of available clean bed linen for women once they had given birth and were dealing with lochia, were disturbing and commonplace features. There were several instances of women who had had caesarean sections with infected wounds, sharing beds with their young babies. The only pain relief these women had was hot water bottles.

Ante-natal Care

Hospital staff confirmed that there was a growing trend of women arriving in Ireland in the second and third trimesters, and even very late arrivals, sometimes within days or even hours of giving birth. These women have very specific needs. They had undertaken extremely long journeys, often involving long plane journeys while close to the end of their pregnancies, and as a result are vulnerable physically at least as much as emotionally. Hospital staff commented that for women arriving at 38 weeks or more, there is seldom time to do more than initiate blood tests and the care routine that is vital for a woman so close to birth. Their social support needs may well remain completely unassessed. The blood work is vital to identify their physical care needs during labour and the puerperium, and can also determine additional needs such as treatment and support for HIV and Hepatitis C. These results can be available within a matter of hours. But with some sexually transmitted diseases, such as syphilis, test results can take anywhere from eight days to three weeks. So there is a risk that, for a tiny number of women, they may already have given birth and moved on from their temporary accommodation by then and yet need special medical intervention and treatment.

With the exception of programme refugees, women reported the following problems in trying to attend for ante-natal care:

- Difficulties in travelling there, including cost

- Arranging childcare

- Being unaccompanied by partner or friend

- Poor health, being too exhausted and stressed

- Language support.

There were no special ante-natal classes or sessions for asylum-seeking women and none of the women had attended the general hospital-based classes.

Experiencing Birth

On the whole, most women managed to negotiate the difficulties of a foreign maternity service, including the hospitals, with some confidence about the level of physical care they received. Communications with staff during ante-natal visits and the labour itself about procedures appeared to be satisfactory on the whole, despite language difficulties. However, staff members working under pressure of time and inadequate resources did result in less than adequate communication, which in turn was perceived as a form of racism, as experienced by the women themselves:

> When I was crying and in pain, I got no sympathy from the
> staff, I had to ask, "Is it because I am black?"

Good standards of physical care did not prevent women from
having fearful and anxious emotions during birth:

> I was afraid, I was so afraid. My mother was not here. No one
> was here. I was afraid this child would die. I was so happy
> when I came out of hospital with my baby. I was crying all the
> time from happiness.

Breastfeeding

Most asylum-seeking women come from countries where breastfeeding is a given for women. But continued breastfeeding is dependent on a materially and socially supportive context. Barriers
to successful breastfeeding include exhaustion, stress and poor
diet. Some women reported feeling under undue pressure from
hospital staff to breastfeed because of assumptions regarding their
ethnicity that this was "what African women do naturally".

Coping without the Extended Family

It was especially evident from the women that family members
play a huge part in the social support system of pregnant and new
mothers. Yet most of the respondents were here without that family network. Despite the emotional pain of often giving birth on
their own with no immediate family member with them or even
in the country, and with difficult and sad memories of events,
family and children they had left behind, women were coping as
best they could:

> We were lonely and alone. We didn't know how to manage
> and I was very weak. . . . When I came here, with no family
> and the climate was so different, I couldn't stop vomiting for
> the first few days I was here.

The Future for Women Asylum-Seekers

Refugee and asylum-seeking women leave hospital with a new
baby and a future marked by insecurity in terms of relationships,

accommodation and income. The impact on women is considerable. One woman who had left her husband and two children behind her in Nigeria and who had no other family here, save her
new baby, said bluntly: "We don't know what is going to happen.
The future is bleak." Another woman expressed it this way:

> I'm worried about taking care of myself and my baby. I think
> about that all the time. Where will they move me? If they
> don't put you in good accommodation, how can you do your
> best? I wonder all the time to myself how will I manage.

Labour and Birth

Most women were coming from countries with highly medicalised
systems of hospital birth but often with poorly trained personnel
and poor equipment. Women were also less willing to state their
needs and wishes. For example, a woman who eventually required
blood after a difficult delivery where there were placental problems and heavy bleeding, was amazed that a family member did
not have to give blood first before she could have what she
needed, as would have been the practice at home. So in that sense,
Dublin hospitals appeared to them excellent. The issue of reassurance is key in all of this and it is vital for maternity care staff to
bear this in mind when dealing with refugee women. Hospital
staff could not overcome the problems of sadness and isolation. It
is critical for hospital staff to develop active procedures to respond
to the often very precarious emotional situations of these women.
Empathic delivery of care, regardless of the explanations about
specific routines, and perhaps even regardless of the routines
(which in Ireland as demonstrated in this book are highly medicalised), may be the most important factor for women.

Emotional Needs and Practical Support Needs

The importance of social support during the maternity period has
been demonstrated in this book. For refugee and asylum-seeking
women, the isolation was terribly striking and worrying. For
women whose partners were with them, it was somewhat reduced.

As explored in Chapter Seven, in Ireland the public health nurse is required to call only once during the ten days after childbirth. The women interviewed in this study for the most part reported having left behind very strong systems of social support. Women were used to expecting and receiving high levels of support from their own communities and, in particular, the women of all generations in those communities. They felt particularly isolated and lonely during pregnancy and following childbirth. In 2002, the National Maternity Hospital employed an additional one and a half social workers to deal with the increased demands on their services, which they viewed as directly related to the complexities of life for this new population of mothers attending the hospital.

Maternity care services in Ireland in the community are very limited at present. In line with the recommendations of the 1994 *Report of the Maternity and Infant Review Group*, it would seem appropriate that where possible public health nurses would make contact with women prior to delivery. This would extend support during the ante-natal period. Women who have settled in Ireland could be trained as link workers/advocates and be employed as such. Similarly, family support workers could be more readily available to asylum-seeking and refugee women and in the long term women who had been refugees themselves could be trained and employed in this capacity. This would provide practical support in the absence of an extended family and it would also be seen to help local integration in the period after birth. There would appear to be a need for a special support unit for third trimester pregnancies, special workers in reception centres to help them link in with hospitals, GPs and community public health nurses before birth. It is possible that supportive accommodation be developed for mothers and babies during pregnancy and the first months of the baby's life.

The Community Mothers Programme, already in existence in some community care areas, could be adapted to meet the needs of refugee women by harnessing the expertise of mothers who have been in Ireland for a while who have experienced the asylum process themselves. Similarly, in the health centre where women attend with their children for developmental check-ups and nurse advisory clinics, which is a potential meeting place for women, supportive groups could be developed if pressures of time and space allowed. NGOs already working with refugee and asylum-seekers could be facilitated and funded to provide such services.

Despite all the practical and emotional difficulties women asylum-seekers face, they demonstrate great competence, adaptability and resilience. While women who come to Ireland as asylum-seekers and refugees experience reasonable health care, especially when compared with the situations from which they have fled, they suffer deeply from the marginalisation that is imposed on them by virtue of their uncertain legal status. The challenge to our services is to respond to this range of need by fully acknowledging the vulnerabilities of this special group of pregnant women and new mothers, and seeking to compensate in practical support terms.

CONCLUSION

Institutional racism can be overt, covert, intentional and unintentional. Institutionalised racism can result from an intention to provide a service which will treat all people the same in attempting to be equitable, but this may in fact fail to acknowledge diversity and difference. This can be remedied with cultural awareness training, orientation and sensitised race relations sessions for staff. Amongst writers on multicultural societies, there is a strong argument that each ethnic group has special and specific needs in relation to health. But paradoxically, it is also argued that what is needed is not a "cultural" approach but one based on need, which in turn stems from the experiences of these groups in contemporary societies. There is a requirement for a system to be set in place which can rapidly collate and re-direct information as new needs arise from ethnic groups. In the Irish setting, such challenges also apply in relation to meeting the maternity needs of Traveller women.

Chapter Nine

DISABILITY AND MATERNITY

People with disabilities are the neglected citizens of Ireland. . . . On the eve of the 21st century, many of them suffer intolerable conditions because of outdated social and economic policies and unthinking public attitudes (*The Commission on the Status of People with Disabilities*, Department of Justice, Equality and Law Reform, 1996: 5).

This book is concerned with the social and medical models of maternity as experienced in Irish society. In respect of disabled women, there are similar models put forward in order to analyse disability. There exists a medical model, also known as the individual model, and the personal tragedy model where the person is expected to adjust to wider society. There is the social oppression model, which places the onus on society to adjust to the disabled person. The disabled are viewed as an oppressed group and are prevented from achieving their full potential from the structures, ideologies and discourses of society. Morris, a disabled mother herself, argues that, like women, disabled people's politicisation has its roots in the assertion that "the personal is political, that our personal experiences of being denied opportunities are not to be explained by our bodily limitations (our impairments) but by the social, environmental, and attitudinal barriers which are a daily part of our lives" (1996: 5). These are the focus of this chapter in relation to pregnancy and maternity in Ireland.

DISABLED WOMEN OR WOMEN WITH DISABILITIES: THE DEBATE

Fawcett examines what she calls the contested topic of disability. She argues that the "individualist model" or medical model and the social model can be "regarded as forming opposing parts of the same frame" (2000: 16). She notes how Oliver in 1993 originally used the term "individual model" to refer to the medical model. These she argues were followed by the psychological, charity and administrative models. These, Fawcett argues, all have been influenced by biological determinism and focus on medically orientated "cure and care" agendas (2000: 16–17). She suggests that the "medical model" has over time come to be used as the "medicalisation" of disability (2000: 17). Oliver, describing the origins of the social model of disability, indicates that in the UK it was associated with the emergence of the Disablement Income Group, which later became the Disability Alliance and the Union of Physically Impaired Against Segregation. UPIAS published *The Key Fundamental Principles of Disability*. In an edited version of the document Oliver writes:

> In our view it is society, which disables physically impaired people. Disability is something imposed on top of our impairments by the way we are unnecessarily isolated and excluded from full participation in society. Disabled people are therefore an oppressed group in society. To understand this it is necessary to grasp the distinction between the physical impairment and the social situation, called "disability" of people with such impairment (1996: 220).

Oliver (1996) uses the work of T.H. Marshall on citizenship to link civil, social and political rights to disability. Crow differentiates between the social model of disability and the medical model of disability, but importantly, she focuses on the place of "impairment" in this debate:

> . . . the social model shifts the focus from impairment onto disability, using this term to refer to disabling social, environmental and attitudinal barriers rather than lack of ability.

> Thus, while impairment is the functional limitation(s) which affect a person's body, disability is the loss or limitation of opportunities resulting from direct and indirect discrimination. Social change — the removal of disabling barriers — is the solution to the disadvantages we experience (1996: 207).

The medical model on the other hand centres on impairment as the cause of experience and disadvantage and impairment as the focus for intervention (1996: 207). She refers to the World Health Organisation definitions of Impairment, Disability and Handicap as:

- **Impairment**: any loss or abnormality of psychological, physiological, or anatomical structure or function

- **Disability**: Any restriction or lack (resulting from impairment) of ability to perform an activity in the manner or within the range considered normal for a human being

- **Handicap:** A disadvantage for a given individual, resulting from an impairment or disability, that limits or prevents fulfilment of a role that is normal, depending on age, sex, social or cultural factors for that individual (United Nations Division for Economic and Social Information, 1983: 3).

Crow suggests that, with the medical model of disability, "a person's functional limitations (impairments) are the root cause of any disadvantages experienced and these disadvantages can therefore only be rectified by treatment or cure" (Crow: 1996: 208). She argues that impairments are not always irrelevant. They are not always neutral or positive. "How can it be when pain, fatigue, depression and chronic illness are constant facts of life for many of us?" (Crow, 1996: 209). She argues convincingly:

> . . . this silence prevents us from dealing effectively with the difficult aspects of impairment. Many of us remain frustrated and disheartened by pain, fatigue, depression and chronic illness, including the way they prevent us from realising our potential or railing fully against disability (our experience of exclusion and discrimination; many of us fear for our futures

with progressive or additional impairments; we mourn past activities that are no longer possible for us; we are afraid we may die early or that suicide may seem our only option; we desperately seek some effective medical intervention; we feel ambivalent about the possibilities of our children having impairments; and we are motivated to work for the prevention of impairments;. Yet our silence about impairment has made many of these taboo and created a whole new series of constraints of our self-expression (Crow, 1996: 210–211).

SPECIFIC NEEDS IN RELATION TO MATERNITY

In relation to pregnancy and maternity, such issues have to be considered. All women, as they progress through the maternity period experience tiredness and discomfort. Many others will find themselves debilitated by morning sickness or more serious complications like raised blood pressure. During pregnancy, labour and delivery, the woman experiences physiological changes. How these are experienced will depend on the general physical health of each individual woman. Hence any "impairment" needs to be considered in this context. In the postpartum period, women are tired, are recovering from the nine months of pregnancy and the exhausting experience of childbirth when they have to come to terms with caring for a new baby and for some mastering the art of breastfeeding. This all places increased emotional and physical demands on the new mother.

French indicates that the ways in which people experience their disability depends on "many interacting factors including social status, personality, personal history and environment" (1994b: 17). Other important variables include: the point in life at which the impairment is acquired; the visibility of the impairment; the comprehensibility of the impairment to others and the presence or absence of illness (French, 1994b: 17). These are all very salient points which need to be addressed in relation to maternity.

Begum indicates that there has traditionally been a tendency to view disabled people as one homogenous group, to the neglect of gender. She suggests that "the dual oppression of sexism and

handicapism places disabled women in an extremely marginal-
ized position" (1992: 70). She notes how class, race, sexuality and
type of disability will influence our experiences. She argues that
the concerns of disabled women strike at the core of both the
feminist and disability rights movements. This is echoed by Fine
and Asch, who remark:

> To be male in our society is to be strong, assertive and inde-
> pendent; to be female is to be weak, passive and dependent,
> the latter conforming to the social stereotypes of the disabled.
> For both categories the disabled women inherits ascriptions of
> passivity, and weakness (1988: 11).

Waddell (1992) talks of a need to challenge attitudes towards
people with disabilities, arguing that "a natural progression for a
woman from accepting and developing herself as a sexual being,
is making a decision as to whether or not to have a family. The
decision is based on many of the same concepts as those for able-
bodied couples" (1992: 7). According to Morris, "the physical act
of giving birth does not in itself determine either the nature of the
relationship between mother and child or the effect on the other's
lifestyle or life chances" (1994: 207). These will be determined by
many different factors such as the general social status of mothers,
the material consequences of having a child, the involvement of
men in parenting, the availability of help with childcare, employment opportunities for women with children (1994: 208). In a
study of 36 women with a variety of disabilities, Rogers and
Matsumura recommends that "the mother with disabilities be
seen primarily as a pregnant woman — both in her own mind and
in the mind of her physician" (1991: 46). They quote one woman
who said, "treat me as a woman first and then secondly as a
woman with a disability" (1991: 46). They make four recommendations to disabled women and to the professionals working with
them:

• Take a positive approach to pregnancy and disability

- The disabled mother-to-be should be seen primarily as a pregnant woman, both in her own mind and in the mind of the physician

- Use a team approach to pregnancy and birth

- Use sensitivity, education and careful planning as the means to achieve the best possible outcome (1991: 49).

Rogers and Matsumura (1991) suggest that in deciding whether or not to have a child, the woman should be encouraged to consider the following: self-image, interaction between pregnancy and disability, the possibility of having disabled children, parenting, the cost of having a child, motherhood and marriage and combining career and family. They indicate that "all women with physical disabilities are likely to have increased mobility problems and associated fatigue in late pregnancy" (1991: 57). They suggest that "specific problems sometimes associated with disability . . . should be evaluated before conception . . . also, some disability symptoms may be worsened by pregnancy symptoms". Other possible problems arise in relation to breastfeeding, medication, physical limitations, exacerbation of disability and prevention of fatigue (1991: 333–334). Morris states that "twenty of us have had children following paralysis (and three were pregnant when injured). For most of us, this has been a positive experience, and we have emphasised what is possible rather than the limitations experienced" (1989: 133).

Begum, in a study of disabled women's experiences of GPs, sees the barriers as accessibility and attitude. To improve women's access to GP services:

> . . . communication, information and a recognition of disabled women's expertise in their own health needs were identified as key factors in ensuring that the contact between disabled women and GPs is constructive (1992: 191).

Morris (1995: 68) suggests that the disability movement's concept of independent living raises particular issues for disabled women.

She indicates that independent living is about having a choice and control over the assistance needed, rather than necessarily doing everything for yourself. Morris (1995) describes the philosophy of the independent living movement as:

- All human life is of value

- Anyone, regardless of impairment, is capable of making choices

- People who are disabled by society's reaction to physical, sensory and intellectual impairment and emotional distress have the right to assert control over their own lives

- Disabled people have the right to participate fully in society.

However, gender inequalities may also inhibit the choice and control that women have in their lives. She writes of "our rights to have a home of our own, to live with those we love and who love us, our rights to have children and to bring them up in the way that non-disabled women take for granted" (1995: 72). She refers to the Independent Living Movement as embracing the whole range of human and civil rights (1995: 74). This includes the right to be a parent. She looks at the concepts of dependence and independence and states that "in Western culture to be dependent is to be subordinate, to be subject to the control of others". On the other hand, to be independent means:

> . . . the ability to do things for oneself, to be self-supporting, self-reliant. . . . When physical impairment means that there are things that someone cannot do for themselves, daily living tasks which they need help with, the assumption is that that person is "dependent" (1995: 74).

She refers to the need for personal assistance as having been translated into a need for "care" in the sense of a need to be looked after; then the "carer" becomes the person in charge, the person in control (1995: 74). She explains how control over personal assistance "enables the expression of individuality and from this then flows the assertion of disabled people's human rights and their status as citizens" (1995: 75). Morris acknowledges that disability is more complex for women because of a lack of economic independence and sexism.

Research conducted by the Maternity Alliance in Britain (1993a), *Mother's Pride and Other Prejudice,* shows that parents may be reluctant to ask for support because of the attitudes of health and social service professionals. Some mothers expressed a fear of having their child removed from them. They believed that their abilities as parents were questioned. Some respondents expressed their concern at the tendency of helpers to take over the care of their children instead of supporting them and therefore a need to rely on family members, including children, was created by the way that resources are allocated and organised by social service departments . Fine and Asch remind us that "problems in mothering for disabled women are not limited to the medical aspects of reproduction" (1988: 22).

In the Irish context, the report of the Maternity and Infant Care Scheme Review Group (Department of Health, 1997b) states that while it feels that services provided under the Scheme meets the needs of mothers generally there are some groups who have special needs which should be dealt with as flexibly and adequately as possible: "It is important that services reflect the requirements of women with special needs" (1997b: 35). It refers in particular to single mothers, Travellers, "people with a mental handicap", people with a physical disability and people with significant illnesses such as AIDS and HIV. In relation to these groups, the Review Group recommends that:

- Service providers should ensure that the requirements of women with special needs are recognised and dealt with as flexibly as possible

- Care should be planned jointly with the woman and any appropriate specialists according to her individual needs and wishes, the same as any other pregnant women

- Women with special needs should be provided with support services, including home help, as required.

This is a very inadequate treatment of such an important aspect of the maternity service. It lumps together several groups of women who have very different yet specific additional needs to the majority of the population of women accessing the maternity services. It ignores such pertinent issues as those raised by Quin and Redmond (1999) and Walsh and Heller (2002). Quin and Redmond (1999: 147), defining intellectual disability, present data from the National Intellectual database, which shows that in 1996, 26,694 individuals with intellectual disability were living in Ireland, with a prevalence rate of 7.57/1,000 total population. They define a person with an intellectual disability as having:

> . . . greater than average difficulty in learning and has a below average intelligence. This results in a delayed or incomplete development of a person's mind and presents difficulties for the individual in acquiring adequate social competencies and self-help skills.

Redmond completed a study in which she interviewed 78 parents of teenage girls with an intellectual disability. She indicates that their largest existing fear was that their daughter would be sexually exploited or would become pregnant (1996: 11).

Walsh and Heller (2002) refer to "intellectual disability" to express a state of functioning manifested before adulthood characterised by substantial limitations in the individual's present cognitive and adaptive functioning (2002: 2–3). They argue that "human rights have supplanted welfare-based policies as the basis for actions related to the lives of persons with disabilities" (2002: 11). This is voiced by the EU in its 1998 policy document (Commission of the European Communities, 1998) where Walsh says it "endorses a rights-based model of disability to replace a traditional model based on providing enough care to compensate people whose impairments left them at a disadvantage" (2002: 11) Today, human rights are expressed as equal opportunities for all citizens, particularly those with disabilities, to take part fully in all aspects of everyday life in their own societies.

In a review of literature on parenting and intellectual disability, Parish (2002: 103) notes that in relation to investigations of parenting by women with intellectual disabilities, the focus is on "the attributes or individual situation of the mothers or their children, ignoring the larger environment in which they lived". Parish suggests that, while in the past mothering by ID women was frowned upon because of a concern with the genetic material, nowadays "opposition and concern about mothers with intellectual disabilities is related to their supposed incompetence and deficiencies in providing appropriate parenting to their children" (2002: 107).

In 1999, the first progress report on the implementation of the recommendations of the Commission on the Status of People with Disabilities was published. *Towards Equal Citizenship* (Department of Justice, Equality and Law Reform, 1999) is an attempt to assess progress achieved since the 1996 report. While there would appear to have been progress made in relation to legislation, structures and organizations, specific progress in relation to meeting the needs of disabled women during the maternity period is absent from the report. This is due in part to the fact that pregnant women did not receive any substantial attention in the Commission Report of 1996. Recommendation 132 of the Report was in relation to maternity units and the proposal was that maternity hospitals should liaise with community services in relation to follow-up care of all infants. There is no mention of the fact that the woman using the maternity hospital may be there as a pregnant woman. It does, however, acknowledge that the ante-natal and post-natal care offered through the public health service is often inaccessible and inappropriate for disabled women (Recommendation 314). Acknowledging that there is a need for more specific services such as the ante-natal classes with a sign interpreter at the Rotunda, it states there are insufficient examples of such initiatives. The 1999 Report indicates that the matter is being pursued by the Department of Health and Children in the context of the ongoing development of ante-natal and post-natal care. Having looked in detail at the complexities of such care, this seems a very cursory treatment of such an important issue.

Personal communication with the three maternity hospitals under study in this book confirmed that the approach taken towards disabled women during the maternity period is a multi-disciplinary one. Like all other women who attend for ante-natal care, disabled women's medical needs are assessed. If there are any additional support needs, the social work team in the hospital is contacted with a view to organising the appropriate services. It would appear that in the postpartum period, once the woman is discharged from hospital, family, friends and NGOs are key providers of personal care and support services. Recommendation 401 of the Commission Report (1996) is that the National Disability Authority should conduct and commission research on disability issues and that adequate funding be made available to extend the scope and volume of such research.

This chapter has raised some issues which need urgent attention in the Irish context. An exploration of maternity services in Ireland from the consumer's perspective is necessary to assess the extent to which they are meeting the needs of disabled women. This would be worth doing in the context of Wilding's model of care as introduced in the previous chapter, in which he identified four key attributes which can be measured in the search for quality care: accessibility, acceptability, effectiveness and openness in terms of aims, objectives, communications and practice.

Chapter Ten

DRUG USE AND PREGNANCY

This book has argued from the beginning that pregnancy and maternity are just one aspect of a woman's life and a woman's needs during the maternity period are part of a complex web. This is particularly relevant to the woman who is abusing or has abused drugs. This book is concerned with the social and medical models of maternity as experienced in Irish society. In respect of women who abuse drugs, there is a parallel dichotomy in relation to access to services. There exists a medical model, which is concerned with the medical treatment of women in this category. There is a social model, which views the women holistically in the context of their biographical and social contexts. Writing on the development of treatment models of addiction, Shea indicates that two distinct treatment models existed historically. These were "abstinence and maintenance" (1991: 15). She argues that the appearance of Acquired Immune Deficiency Syndrome (AIDS) ushered in a third model that was "harm minimization". This is particularly relevant to the pregnant woman as the health of the developing fetus and the new baby becomes an issue. Some of these issues are explored in this chapter.

The age profile of drug users coincides with women's childbearing years. In general, women drug users suffer from more medical problems than their male counterparts (Bourke, 1997; Farrell, 2001). They are at increased risk of sexually transmitted diseases (STDs), hepatitis, anaemia, high blood pressure, urinary tract infections, gynaecological and dental problems. All of these are health factors which are directly relevant to pregnancy.

These women are more likely to engage in risk behaviour, to be living with a partner who uses drugs and to suffer from health problems which are related to drug use. However, women are more likely to acknowledge their problems and to access help. O'Brien and Dillon (2001: 56) indicate that the typical heroin-user is a young, unemployed, early school leaver living in a socially and economically deprived area. Farrell (2001) reviews some early studies carried out in Dublin in relation to pregnancy and drug use. She concludes that opiate-dependent women when pregnant are a high-risk medical category with complex psychological and social problems. They tend to be young, poorly educated, regular tobacco smokers and from socially deprived areas. She indicates that these women have a high level of psychological difficulty and, in common with international findings, dysfunctional family life rather than poverty seems to be one of the most significant predisposing factors to drug use. Murphy-Lawless, in her study conducted in North Inner City Dublin, quotes one health board worker who states in relation to drug users:

> There is a very high rate of unemployment. Some of them are functionally illiterate. In some streets and blocks of flats, there is 50 per cent unemployment, usually intergenerational, families which are termed dysfunctional; there are big alcohol problems as well. Parents are often very young themselves and not very mature . . . there are quite a lot of teenage pregnancies, and they are getting younger. The sense of achievement and pride in their beautiful children is an important aspect. However, as they get older and get into mischief, frustration grows, and the parents are missing out on their own adolescence (2002: 46).

DRUG ABUSE IN IRELAND

In Ireland, information on problem drug use is collected by the National Drug Treatment Reporting System (NDTRS). It is an epidemiological database on treated drug misuse. It was established in 1990 in the Greater Dublin area and in 1995 was extended to cover other areas. As the most serious drug problems in

Ireland to date have occurred mainly in Dublin and this book has concentrated primarily on the three main maternity units there, the same emphasis will be placed here. Almost all of the 5,380 people who received treatment in the EHB during 1999 were resident there. Treatment is defined as "any activity which aims to ameliorate the psychological, medical or social state of individuals who seek help for their drug problems" (Drug Misuse Research Division, 2002: 1). This definition would seem to combine both the social and medical models of care. The ratio of males to females treated in 1999 was 67:33. Trends show an increase in the misuse of opiates. Of those who used heroin, 71 per cent injected the drug. In 1999 of those injecting, 57 per cent had shared equipment. Poly-drug use is the commonest type of drug abuse in Dublin.

DRUG USE: SPECIFIC NEEDS IN RELATION TO MATERNITY

Bourke indicates that low self-esteem is a problem in female drug users and states that "this is a serious issue about which we need to be pro-active" (1997: 29). Many of her recommendations are important in the context of maternity as they are directed at General Practitioners and indicate the range of issues which arise for this group of mothers. These include difficulty in accessing programmes as well as difficulty remaining in programmes. This is very relevant in relation to ante-natal care and ante-natal education as often those who have most to benefit from such programmes fail to attend (Enkin, 2000). They may have little support from a partner and may in fact be under tremendous pressure from a partner who may also be a drug user. Social support is crucially important for the new mother, particularly a first-time mother. When there is no familial support either from partner or the extended family, support from the statutory sector is crucial. This is underdeveloped in Ireland.

Sloan and O'Connor (1998) indicate that the absence of periods (amennorrhoea) caused by opiate use is often understood by opiate-addicted women to equate with infertility. This is incorrect. The problem is compounded by polysubstance abuse. Sloan and O'Connor argue that, because of their low molecular weight, heroin and other opiates pass easily through the placental barrier. Maternal drug use during pregnancy causes medical, neurological, cardiovascular and respiratory complications, in addition to an increased incidence of infectious diseases. Sloan and O'Connor also indicate that higher rates of mortality and morbidity among babies have been reported, as have abortion, prematurity, IUGR, stillbirth, congenital abnormalities, abruptio placentae and fetal distress. There is some evidence to show a link with SIDS. The neonatal symptoms of withdrawal from opiates includes hypertonicity, irritability, convulsions, disturbed sleep patterns and poor feeding. Sloan and O'Connor (1998) argue that:

> . . . complications of maternal drug use, both for the mother and the child must therefore be seen in the context of the drug taking environment, which is invariably a stressful one, with associated poverty, poor nutrition and concomitant use of cigarettes.

Milner et al. (1999) completed a 12-month review of infants admitted with neonatal abstinence syndrome to a neonatal intensive care unit in Dublin. In the study of 43 infants, the average maternal age was 24.6 (18–34 years). In the 12-month period studied, 8.3 per cent of the total bed occupancy and 3.5 per cent of all paediatric admissions were due to NAS at the Rotunda.

Siney (1995, 1997, 1999) indicates that drug use places women at high risk during pregnancy. Because of the possibility that diagnosis of pregnancy can be delayed there can be a delay in booking for ante-natal care. Fewer ante-natal visits, longer and more frequent hospital admissions can also be common to drug users. Reasons for poor attendance at ante-natal care can be the same as those expressed by the general population (Department of Health, 1997b). These include a perception that it is inaccessible, either geographically and/or administratively. However, barriers specific to the drug addict may include demands on time because of having to finance a drug habit. Another common fear is that the child will be taken into care. With some women, failure to disclose their drug use is a barrier to attending for ante-natal care.

This is why Siney argues that it is important that ante-natal care be provided in a relaxed way so that the woman will be open about her drug use in order to receive appropriate care and advice in relation to booking for appointments, paediatric services and withdrawal (1997: 134). This will help women who otherwise fear they may be judged as unfit mothers, that they may be treated differently from other women. She refers to the importance of trust between women who work in the maternity services and also between all professionals who work with drug-using women (1997: 136). The clinical report for the Coombe draws attention to the myths surrounding early disclosure of drug history leading to the implementation of child protection practices (2000: 90). Keogh, in a small study of the social work role in relation to pregnancy and heroin addiction (2002), reviews some of the literature on the subject and concludes that social work with heroin users has generally been approached from a child protection perspective. This has not only resulted in the neglect of the mothers' needs but has also under-utilised the mothers' resilience and resources. She suggests that "feminist social work . . . offers women a more centred and sensitive way of attempting to combine the needs of both the mother and the unborn baby" (2002: 39). Interestingly, Keogh suggests that:

> . . . the interviews with the social workers revealed many of the same concerns as those with the women in the treatment centre. These were the relationship and trust in the social worker/client relationship and the brevity of the interventions (2002: 45).

Shea indicates that drug users are labelled negatively and female drug users "are treated particularly judgementally and are seen to be even more reckless and blameworthy than their male counterparts" (1991: 22). She quotes from the Drugs, Alcohol, Women Now Symposium held in 1980, arguing that these same attitudes continue to prevail:

> Women who use illicit drugs are beyond the moral pale. Their behaviour goes against people's expectations of the feminine

and is typified as selfish, deviant, criminal, etc. Greater horror is expressed at women users than men. This is particularly clear from the enormous concern about mothers, never fathers, using drugs.

Farrell (2001) summarises the main barriers for women accessing services as lack of childcare services and fear of being labelled "an unfit mother".

Siney (1997: 140) presents guidelines on the management of pregnant substance abusers. She also provides guidelines for the management of their babies (1997: 142) and "pointers for practice", summarising that "the only way to encourage both registered and non-registered drug users to identify and attend for antenatal care is to develop an attractive, low-key, women-centred service that guarantees confidentiality and sympathetic care" (1997: 144). Acknowledging the importance of normalisation, she states that "all body fluids from all women should be considered to be risky to staff, and therefore clinical practices should be of the highest standard in every case and not just where a woman is known to be HIV positive or an intravenous drug user" (1997: 136).

The European Monitoring Centre for Drugs and Drug Addictions (EMCDDA) annual report (2000) states that over 60 per cent of female addicts support their habit through the drug industry and suggest that "pregnancy is perhaps the most emotive aspect of narcotic drug abuse. Expectant drug addicts require a particularly high level of intervention and support". In all EU countries, pregnant women are fast-tracked into drug treatment programmes. In Ireland there are three Drug Liaison Midwives. These are all in the ERHA and are attached to the three maternity hospitals under study in this book. Drug Liaison Midwives are paid by the drug service. The model developed in the ERHA is based on that developed at the Liverpool Women's Hospital (Siney, 1999). The midwife has the status of a staff nurse/clinical nurse specialist and carries a caseload of 40 at any one time. In the ERHA, the woman attends the drug clinic for an initial assessment. The nurse in the clinic is the initial point of contact. The woman undergoes a very comprehensive health check. The DLM meets with the medical social worker in the maternity hospital and has permission from the mother to release all information. Urine testing takes place twice a week. There is also a liaison HIV nurse in Our Lady's Hospital for Sick Children, Crumlin. In the Coombe, there is a social worker, family support worker and drug social worker. In an interview with the first drug liaison midwife in the ERHA, it was expressed to this author that for a certain cohort of dependent addicts, becoming pregnant will provide the first entry to treatment for women otherwise unlikely to present to drug treatment services. Hence, the first ante-natal appointment can provide the opportunity for the first identification of dependence on drugs. However, other women will continue to abuse drugs despite their pregnancy.

Bourke lists the most important issue for pregnant drug users: it is safer for the baby if the mother is not using street drugs. If the mother is on methadone maintenance she has more opportunity for better ante-natal care and shorter hospital stays are noted for the baby (1997: 30). If the baby is maintained on methadone it will not affect the baby in utero; if detoxifying, the mother should be detoxed in the mid-trimester. This is because detoxification in the first trimester leads to a higher incidence of miscarriage. Detoxification in the last trimester shows a higher incidence of early delivery. The postpartum period is a period of increased risk of relapse. This in Ireland was reported to be as high as 50 per cent (Keenan et al., 1993). The benefits of methadone include:

- Cyclical craving for opiates is eliminated.

- Potential for infection via adulterants, contaminants or shared needles is reduced.

- Maternal nutrition is improved and criminal activity reduced. Women are more amenable to attending ante-natal care and accessing psychosocial reports. They can prepare and plan for mothering and rehabilitation.

- Dosage depends on history and motivation of the individual.

Keenan et al. conclude that mothers in methadone treatment programmes have been shown to have longer gestational periods, larger babies, and fewer obstetric complications, and conclude that low dose methadone therapy throughout pregnancy is therefore widely advocated. Sloan and O'Connor (1998) indicate that street drugs can lead to increased risk of HIV, Hepatitis B (HBV) and Hepatitis C (HCV) and also possible risk of STD (through prostitution).

PREGNANCY AND HIV

Clarke et al. (2001a) indicate that injecting drug users (IDUs) represent 41.6 per cent of the total cohort of HIV-infected patients in Ireland. They indicate that while there was an overall reduction in the incidence of HIV infection in Ireland between 1990 and 1998, between January 1999 and December 2000 referrals to the GUIDE clinic, the Genito-Urinary Medicine and Infectious Disease Clinic at St James's Hospital, the largest tertiary centre for HIV, increased dramatically. The number of new HIV diagnoses in IDU increased fivefold between 1995 and 2000. Forty-four per cent of patients diagnosed were under 22 years of age. They summarise that there is a need to focus on improving health education to reduce both sexual and needle-sharing practices. If HIV status is known, measures can be taken to reduce the risk of vertical spread by as much as 50 per cent. Farrell (2001) indicates how routine screening for HIV was introduced in 1999. She refers to a 1999 Department of Health and Children report which indicates that 54 per cent of registered female AIDS cases were IDU-related. Butler and Woods (1992) demonstrate that women who were HIV positive tend to see their own health problems as less important than those of their families. The clinical report of the NMH (2000) indicates the social work department offers pre-test counselling to women who perceive themselves at risk of contacting HIV (page 123). Counselling is provided to women already diagnosed with HIV. This is as a result of the 1998 National AIDS Strategy Report.

Almost all women who are known to be HIV positive are of childbearing age. Pregnancy does not appear to affect progression of HIV diseases for women who are asymptomatic. Once the disease has progressed to where a woman's immune system is compromised, progression can be rapid during pregnancy. HIV does not affect the outcome of pregnancy. There is no increased risk of spontaneous abortion or prematurity. All babies born to mothers with HIV will have antibodies at birth. These usually disappear by about 15 months if the baby is not infected. Babies born to HIV-infected mothers who have received no antiretroviral therapy should be started on zidovudine syrup within 12 to 24 hours of birth (Siney, 1999: 99). There is less than one in four chance of the baby being infected. Vertical transmission can occur transplacentally, during labour, at delivery and breastfeeding. Bourke (1997: 31) states that HIV women should be discouraged from breastfeeding. Breastfeeding doubles the risk to 30 per cent. Weingrad Smith and Tully (2001: 431) identifies this, however, as a very controversial issue as recommendations vary between developed and developing countries. Advice from the WHO is that in developing countries, mothers should exclusively breastfeed their infants unless replacement feeding is safe, accessible and affordable. The highest transmission risk seems to be in relation to mixed feedings (WHO, 2001). In this context, it is important to bear in mind that many of the women arriving in Ireland as asylum-seekers and giving birth here may not have full and accurate information in relation to best practice in this regard.

Patchen and Beal (2001: 355) indicate that major advances have been made in relation to care of HIV women who are pregnant: the development of successful regimens for the prevention and treatment of opportunistic infections, the use of combination retroviral therapy and the development of laboratory testing that allows providers to more effectively assess the dynamics of HIV infection and adjust medications accordingly. There are several tests for the presence of the HIV virus in body fluids.

Scarrow (2001) indicates that medical studies endorse delivery by caesarean section to reduce mother to infant (vertical) transmission of HIV. This raises important ethical questions for the attendant physician. The issue of HIV and pregnancy was launched onto the public agenda in Ireland as recently as July 2002 when a High Court judge ordered a woman to have treatment to prevent the transmission of HIV to her unborn child. The woman had refused ante-natal treatment to prevent HIV transmission and also said that she would not give birth in the Coombe Women's Hospital because she did not trust the doctors there. The woman had tested positive for HIV four months earlier when attending an ante-natal clinic. She had agreed to attend a support clinic for HIV sufferers. The judge decided that on birth the child would be made a ward of court, meaning that the court would direct the treatment. He ordered the administration of medication to the child on birth and further medication, therapy and testing and monitoring, as was advised by the Master of the Coombe, Dr Sean Daly. He also said that he would consider an order restraining the woman from breastfeeding the baby, but when told that the woman did not intend to breastfeed he decided there would not be a need for such an order. The orders relating to the treatment of the unborn child were sought by the South Western Area Health Board (SWAHB).

Scarrow (2001: 178) indicates that in addition to caesarean section there are four strategies currently recommended to physicians in relation to the obstetric care of HIV women: universal voluntary HIV counselling and testing of pregnant women; treatment with zidovudine, both to mothers ante-natally and post-natally and to the infants; obstetric management designed to reduce infants' exposure to maternal blood and genital secretions; and avoidance of breastfeeding. Scarrow (2001: 182) presents guidelines aimed at physicians and obstetricians and gynaecologists when counselling a HIV positive woman. She stresses the importance of identifying the decision-maker and of collecting data, establishing facts, identifying all options and evaluating them according to the patient's values and principles, and selecting the course of action best justified.

A subgroup of the Irish Infection Society, consisting of Genito-Urinary Medicine and Infectious Diseases Consultants, has produced guidelines for the optimal management of HIV disease in pregnancy (Clarke, 2001a). They are based on peer-reviewed international data and guidelines. Since 1994, there have been 100 pregnancies to 94 HIV-infected mothers in Ireland. Clarke (2001a) explains how pregnant mothers with HIV attend a designated mother and baby clinic in the adult infectious disease unit at least every one to two months during pregnancy. This is to allow for monitoring of the HIV infection and treatment. Importantly, Clarke (2001) indicates that "the overall management of HIV in pregnancy requires a multidisciplinary approach between adult and paediatric HIV specialists, obstetric services, and often the drug treatment services". She goes on to say that:

> . . . the changing immigrant population in Ireland provides medical, social and cultural challenges for the management of HIV. . . . While the National Guidelines can be used as a model for the management of HIV in pregnancy, ultimately each patient is managed individually, and a unique antenatal, intrapartum, and postpartum path is determined for each patient.

CONCLUSION

The issues raised in this chapter in relation to the maternity needs of drug users and women who are HIV-positive are complex. While the pregnant drug abuser progresses through the maternity period, she needs ante-natal care and education and access to maternity services like other women. Additionally, she will have very specific medical needs. She will also have very specific social support needs. Interestingly, it would appear that the women in question in this chapter have a greater chance of receiving continuity of care than the general population of women. It would also seem that they have a much better chance of benefiting from a unique pregnancy and birth plan suited to the woman's individual needs. They are also fast-tracked within drug treatment services so they may also fare better than their non-pregnant drug-abusing friends. This specific group of women raise very significant challenges for all involved in the provision of maternity services in both a hospital and community setting.

Chapter Eleven

MATERNITY AND THE STATE

If women enter the public sphere as workers then they must
do so on terms similar to men (Lewis, 1992: 164).

Women's three roles — as earners, carers and lifegivers — are
interlinked and the point where they intersect is the very point
where the public and private domains meet and where women
tend to live their lives. In this chapter, these three strands are
brought together and interwoven, that is, the three strands of
women's lives as earners, carers and lifegivers. At the same time,
health policies, labour policies and welfare policies are interwoven in an attempt to elucidate the relationship between the
Irish welfare state and mothers during the "maternity period".
This chapter begins by introducing the concept of "de-
commodification" and returning to the "male breadwinner
model" (Lewis, 1992) in an attempt to understand the gender dimension of the organisation of welfare and labour market policies
in Ireland, which are directly relevant to women as they experience the maternity period.

DE-COMMODIFICATION: MOTHERS AS EARNERS AND CARERS

According to Esping-Andersen, welfare policies permit, encourage or discourage the de-commodification of labour. Esping-
Andersen (1990: 37) defines de-commodification as "the degree to
which individuals or families can uphold a socially acceptable
standard of living independently of market participation". Lewis
(1993) indicates that commodification ensures that human needs

and labour power become commodities and a person's well-being depends on her relationship to the cash nexus. In this situation, Lewis concludes, purchasing power and redistribution are crucial. According to Esping-Andersen's theory, labour power is also a commodity, which implies that people's rights to exist outside the market are at stake. People, as workers, are commodities and captive to powers beyond their control. They are destroyed by events like illness. They are replaceable and easily rendered redundant. Lewis's succinct summary of the perils of commodification ring loud alarm bells for the woman as she progresses through the maternity period. The woman who has negotiated the difficulties of participating in the labour market, while experiencing morning sickness, nausea, exhaustion, a change of shape, size and identity, then has to deal with the major identity shift to motherhood, cope with breastfeeding, bond with her child, learn how to mother and resource accessible and affordable childcare. To what extent is this woman dispensable within the patriarchal constraints of the labour market? This woman is caught in a bind between the patriarchal employment market, patriarchal healthcare and the patriarchal social welfare systems.

Esping-Andersen (1990) claims that de-commodification is a necessary prerequisite for workers' political mobilisation. Lewis (1992) argues that the worker he has in mind is the male worker whose mobilisation also relies on female support. How possible is it for the pregnant women or new mother to become politically mobilised? Cousins refers to:

> The weakness of a transient category of persons with little organisational representation (pregnant women who are not in employment) in the formation of social policy and highlight the extent to which trade union priorities involve their own members rather than welfare recipients generally (and particularly women who are not in employment) (1995: 114–115).

Lewis (1993) argues that de-commodification for women is likely to involve carrying out unpaid caring work. "Welfare dependency" of a woman is likely to involve caring for others. However, the unequal division of unpaid work blurs the division between dependent and independent, commodified and de-commodified. Because women conceive, become pregnant, give birth and nurse babies, they tend to find themselves in the role of carer for their infants. This caring role is prescribed for women in Irish society.

IRELAND AS A MALE BREADWINNER-TYPE STATE

Jane Lewis (1992) presents a theoretical model which deals with the gender dimension of welfare states. In her three-tiered model of welfare states as weak, modified and strong male breadwinner-type states, Lewis categorises Ireland as a strong male breadwinner-type state (Kennedy, 1999). According to Lewis's typology, these states are characterised by low labour participation rates for women, a high incidence of part-time work, underdeveloped childcare, poor maternity entitlements and inequality between husbands and wives in relation to social security. This is a useful model from which to begin analysing mothers' relationship to the labour market and the social welfare system in Ireland, that is, women's role as earner and as carer.

WOMEN AS CARERS

Only women can give birth and only women can breastfeed. These are physiological facts. But caring in our society is socially constructed. In the postpartum period, mothers in Ireland, in general, do most of the caring work. Graham (1983) refers to caring as both an "identity and activity". Mothers give birth and in the period following childbirth they take on the role and identity of principal carer. Mothers take on the physical work of caring. This physical work also has an emotional aspect. Lynch and McLaughlin refer to "love labour" as:

> . . . not like materially productive labour as originally conceived. It is not about the moulding and manipulation of raw materials to create some desired end product. . . . Love labour involves reciprocity in most cases . . . social relations are not one way (1995: 264).

They distinguish between caring for and caring about, and refer to the fact that "caring for" can be commodified and that this is in fact a booming industry. However, caring about is more difficult to commodify, "one cannot provide love on a rational contractual basis like one provides other services" (1995: 261). As Lynch and McLaughlin explain, "one cannot pay someone to love someone else . . . one cannot pay one to hug one's children and pretend that this is 'one's own hug'" (1995: 263). The very nature of love labour, and this is very much the type of work that is involved in caring for infants, especially when the mother has her own demanding emotional, psychological, social and physical needs, renders both parties vulnerable. Nic Ghiolla Phadraig (1994) refers to the vulnerability of the recipient of care, an issue which has become increasingly visible in feminist writing (Morris, 1991). The focus of this book is on the mother, the carer; therefore it is her vulnerability with which we are here primarily concerned. Feminist writers, including Pateman (1988) and Delphy and Leonard (1992), have focused on the exploitative nature of caring work. Yet caring is something that very many women want to do and get the utmost enjoyment, satisfaction and fulfilment from this role (Benn, 1998). The fact that approximately 50,000 Irish women continue to give birth each year is evidence of this.

WOMEN AS EARNERS

Employment is a general prerequisite to independence. Traditionally, the majority of women in Ireland have been denied access to paid employment (Conroy Jackson, 1993, 1997; Smyth, 1997). This is now changing. In the past, mothers had particular difficulty in accessing well-paid full-time employment for a variety of reasons. Women working outside the home need a good standard of accessible, affordable childcare. This has never been available in Ireland. Childcare facilities in Ireland are underdeveloped and there is no tax relief on childcare. Few workplace nurseries are in existence (Ditch et al., 1997). An ideology which postulates that childcare provision is a private issue ensures that Ireland has one of the lowest levels of public childcare in the EU.

The Chambers of Commerce of Ireland in a 2001 study examines the issue of childcare in a labour market context from the employers' perspective. It highlights ongoing labour shortages, despite recent changes in the employment environment. It remarks on the impact that the lack of affordable childcare is having on employers' ability to recruit staff:

> ... given that childcare still tends to be primarily the responsibility of women, the deficit of affordable childcare also raises the issue of equality of opportunity in terms of labour market participation (2001: 2).

It argues that the overall level of funding earmarked for the development of childcare in Ireland needs to be reviewed. While it acknowledges the allocation of €368 million under the National Development Plan and the anti-inflationary package introduced in 2000, it says there is a need for a much greater level of resourcing, arguing that an overall review of funding needs to be accompanied by a long-term strategy for the development and maintenance of the sector. It states that "in order to attract and retain staff, employers need to continue to develop family-friendly arrangements for the workplace. This will pose challenges for small businesses in particular" (2001: 2).

In half of the companies surveyed, women made up 50 per cent or more of employees. In 21 per cent of companies, staff with children aged 12 years or under comprised the majority of the workforce. Respondents in 57 per cent of the companies surveyed were aware of a query or complaint being made by an employee regarding childcare provision in the previous 12 months. Requests for flexible hours (38 per cent), or complaints about the cost of childcare services (33 per cent) were the most common. Thirteen per cent of the companies experienced a situation in the previous 12 months where one or more of the employees resigned their post to care for children. Almost a third of companies (31 per cent) believed that the lack of affordable or available childcare had a negative impact on their ability to recruit or retain staff. Cost (72 per cent), unavailability (65 per cent) and poor quality (13 per cent) were the principal difficulties faced by employees when looking for childcare services (2001: 3). Seventy-two per cent of companies who have employees with children aged 12 or under have some form of family-friendly arrangements in place above those required by law. The most common were part-time (40 per cent), flexi-time (34 per cent), excess unpaid maternity leave (27 per cent) and job-sharing (24 per cent) (2001: 3). Twenty-eight per cent of all the respondents felt that employees had the main responsibility for childcare, while only 21 per cent of the 503 employers interviewed felt that the responsibility should fall to the government. Only 2 per cent believed that the main responsibility for childcare is that of the employer. Forty-nine per cent of those interviewed (employers) believed that responsibility should be split between a combination of employees, government and employers. Tax relief for employees' expenditure on childcare (62 per cent) and employers' expenditure (39 per cent) were the most common suggestions.

While mothers have been hampered in accessing the labour market, they have also had difficulties in accessing vocational training. Cousins, in *Pathways*, his 1996 study of women returners, whom he defines as women who wish to return to the paid labour force after a period of absence due to family responsibilities, highlights some of the difficulties of this particular group in accessing training which would equip them with the necessary skills for participation in the changing labour market. He outlines the practices which have rendered women invisible but also discriminated against women regarding entry to employment and training schemes. Irish women, and particularly mothers, are underrepresented on the live register as a proportion of those claiming unemployment payments. The live register is an important tool, as it determines a person's right to access training schemes, which are a gateway to employment. For women who wish to return to the labour market having spent time caring full-time for children, or mothers entering the labour market for the first time, access to good quality training and education are essential.

Since the 1970s, there have been some improvements regarding women's labour force status. These are most directly related to Ireland's membership of the EU, which has led to the introduction of equality legislation. Factors such as smaller family size, male unemployment and rising house prices ensure that mothers are more likely to seek full-time employment. Since Ireland has experienced an economic boom, there are more employment opportunities for women, particularly in the services sector. However, women are faced with constantly having to reconcile work and family life and, as this book has argued, the roles and demands of physiological motherhood. Hence, an examination of maternity rights will help to clarify the challenges women face as carer, earner and lifegiver and how Irish social policies respond.

It is difficult to statistically estimate women's participation in the labour market, as statistics available from both the live register and the labour force surveys do not give a true picture of women's labour force participation. This is due to under-representation of women in both sources as a result of the systems of reporting (Cousins, 1996). However, looking at labour force statistics on women of childbearing age gives some indication of women's under-representation (CSO, 1997). In the 25 years between 1971 and 1996, the number of women at work grew by 212,000, reaching 488,000 in 1996. There was a growth rate of 23,000 for males over the same period. These changes have particularly involved married women. In 1971, married women accounted for only 14 per cent of the female workforce, whereas in 1996 about half the female workforce were married. In 1996, using ILO statistics, 41.1 per cent of Irish women aged 15 or over were in the labour force, which compares with 58.7 per cent for Denmark, the highest rate in the EU, and 34.6 per cent for Italy, the lowest in the EU (CSO, 1997).

In 1991, a quarter of all mothers — a third of all mothers with one or two dependent children and over one-fifth of all mothers with three or more dependent children — were in the labour force. Overall, slightly more than 36.6 per cent of mothers were in the labour force in 1996, while about 43 per cent of mothers with one or two dependent children were in the labour force. Only 33.2 per cent of mothers with three or more children were in the labour force (CSO, 1997). As family size increases, after two children, mothers' participation in the labour force decreases. In 1996, of 507,700 women in the labour force, 111,000 were engaged in part-time work (CSO, 1997). Women's high representation among part-time workers is partly due to the fact that women in Ireland have to balance their caring responsibilities with paid work with practically no state support in accessing childcare services.

Almost 50 per cent of women living with a husband/partner in a family unit with children were in employment in June–August 2001 compared with 43.6 per cent three years earlier. The most notable increase in employment participation was for mothers in family units where the youngest child was aged 5 to 14. In this category, the percentage in employment increased from 47.3 per cent to 56.2 per cent between mid-1998 and mid-2001 (CSO, 2001).

MATERNITY ENTITLEMENTS

Social welfare policies amount to no less than state organisation of domestic life (Wilson, 1977: 9).

Lewis (1992) indicates that women in strong male breadwinner-type states must enter the labour force on the same basis as their male colleagues. What are the repercussions of this for Irish mothers in the labour market? There was no maternity leave in Ireland until 1981 when it was introduced under the Maternity Protection of Employees Act. This was superseded by the 1994 Maternity Protection Act. In 2001, as a result of the *Report of the Working Group on the Review and Implementation of the Maternity Protection Legislation*, the period of maternity, adoptive and health and safety leave were extended under the Maternity Protection Act, 1994 (Extension of Periods of Leave) Order 2001 and the Adoptive Leave Act, 1995 (Extension of Periods of Leave) Order 2001.

Protective leave is the term used to collectively refer to maternity leave, additional maternity leave, health and safety leave and leave to which the father is entitled. The 1994 Act provided protection to all pregnant employees who had recently given birth or who were breastfeeding. This Act entitled the woman to 14 weeks maternity leave and up to four weeks' unpaid additional maternity leave. The payment of maternity benefit during this time is the responsibility of the Department of Social, Community and Family Affairs. The 1994 Act guaranteed the woman the right to return to work, the right to take time off work to attend ante-natal and post-natal appointments, without loss of pay. This is an important factor in facilitating women's take-up of ante-natal and post-natal healthcare. The Act guaranteed the woman the right to health and safety leave in certain circumstances. This is in accordance with the requirements of the Pregnant Workers Directive (89/391/EEC) adopted by the Council of Europe in 1992. This was an important departure, as it was the first recognition by the state in Ireland that there exists a maternity period, and that this involves pregnancy and lactation as well as labour and delivery. However, leave on health and safety grounds is not necessarily concerned with the health and safety of the mother. Under the 1989 Safety, Health and Welfare at Work Act, the employer is required to conduct a risk assessment in relation to pregnant employees, employees who have recently given birth and employees who are breastfeeding. When a workplace risk to these employees is identified, the employer is required to either remove the risk or to arrange other suitable work. Health and safety benefit is the responsibility of the Department of Social, Community and Family Affairs; however, the employer is responsible for remuneration for the first 21 days of health and safety leave.

Significantly, the 1994 Act recognised the role of the father during the maternity period, but only where the death of the mother occurs within 14 weeks of the birth. Under the Maternity Protection Act, the jobs of both mother and father are protected during leave. The woman has the right not to be dismissed for any pregnancy-related reason from the beginning of pregnancy through to the end of the maternity leave. Mothers in full-time employment are entitled to resume employment with the same employer at the end of maternity leave.

The woman is required to give the employer four weeks' notice prior to commencement of leave, to take at least four weeks prior to the expected date of delivery and four weeks after. The remaining six weeks could be taken as desired. Some women who are in a position to take an additional amount of unpaid leave have the option to take an additional four weeks. They are entitled to 18 weeks' paid leave and 8 weeks' unpaid leave. This also applies to fathers in the event of the death of the mother. Any adopting mother or sole male adopter who commenced adoptive leave on or after the 8th March was entitled to 14 weeks' paid leave plus 8 weeks' unpaid leave.

This book is concerned with mothers as they progress through the maternity period. This includes mothers who may have never experienced pregnancy or childbirth — mothers who have adopted babies. These women, like all mothers, need time to bond with and get to know their babies. While they will not have had the tiredness and sometimes stress of pregnancy, neither will they have had the experience of feeling their baby moving inside them and growing to know their baby in this way. Instead, they will have had the stress of waiting for word and visits from social workers, of always watching the post and waiting for the telephone to ring to bring them news of a different type of expected date of delivery. These mothers too need time and this eventually was allocated to them in 1995 under the Adoptive Leave Act. This Act guaranteed statutory maternity leave for adoptive mothers, on the same basis as that provided to mothers under the 1994 Maternity Protection Act. This was a welcome development. The period of leave was also extended in 2001. The adoptive mother can take 14 weeks, as she is not allowed leave before she adopts the baby. She is also entitled to take an additional eight weeks' unpaid leave.

The maximum possible maternity leave for Irish women is now 26 weeks. This reflects Hinds's observation of maternity leave entitlements in Northern Ireland when she refers to the system in the United Kingdom as "essentially one of unpaid child care leave for women, a system which promotes traditional patterns of domestic responsibility once a reasonable period for childbirth and maternal health has ended" (Hinds, 1991: 7). It also indicates a two-tier system where women who have the financial resources can take the extra eight weeks' unpaid leave.

The time a woman is allowed to take off from work is significant as it dictates such issues as whether or not a woman can breastfeed her baby and when she has to start to wean her baby. This must be analysed in the context of the 1994 National Breastfeeding Policy, presented earlier in this book, which recommended that a target breastfeeding rate of 30 per cent at four months should be reached by the year 2000. The woman who wants to share the early months of her child's life is denied flexibility and choice and in reality is forced to return to work after 18 weeks (or up to 26 weeks if she can afford the option of taking unpaid leave) or to depend on welfare payments or on a male breadwinner. If she returns to work she must pay somebody, usually another mother or a crèche to care for the new baby. Taking this in the context of health policies for mothers, Irish women are extremely vulnerable at this time in their lives. Women in Ireland, under the Maternity and Infant Care Scheme, can only avail of free medical care during pregnancy and for six weeks after delivery. This is totally inadequate for new mothers (Glazener et al., 1995). The lack of support services (statutory) and also familial and emotional support (paternity and parental leave) in reality implies that women must get on with the task of motherhood drawing on very limited fiscal and social supports.

Mr John O'Donoghue, TD, then Minister for Justice, Equality and Law Reform, at the launch of *The Report of the Working Group on the Review and Improvement of the Maternity Protection Legislation*, on 28 February 2001 stated:

> The way forward is to encourage a greater balance between the responsibilities people face at work and at home. It has been recognised at EU level, and indeed, it makes common

sense, that the facilitation of a better balance between work and family responsibilities contributes positively towards the goal of a healthier and happier workforce and ultimately a healthier and happier society.

Parental Leave and Paternity Leave

There is still no legal entitlement to paternity leave in Ireland (except on the death of the mother under the 1994 Maternity Protection Act) although some private companies do provide a very limited amount of paid leave. Thus, there is no official recognition of the important and often crucial role a father has to play in supporting the mother especially around the time of childbirth (as discussed previously). Nor does it recognise the importance of paternity leave in giving the father the opportunity to bond with his new baby and perhaps to support and mind other children at this important time, when they are coming to terms with having a new sibling. This again questions the extent to which Ireland, which this book argues could be classified as a conservative/ corporatist-type society, views women's role as that of carer within the home, while the father is assigned the role of bread-winner, thereby being excused from the more direct caring parental duties within the home. It also brings under scrutiny the principle of subsidiarity, which limits the involvement of the state in service provision, laying responsibility on the family. The family in this instance has a very gendered meaning, as there is no facility for the father to take paid leave to support the mother in her own right as well as in sharing responsibility for care of the new infant, at the time of childbirth.

Parental leave is an important issue, and one which the EU has recognised. The Council of Social Affairs Ministers adopted a Directive on Parental Leave in 1996 (96/34/EC). This was the first measure to be agreed under the social protocol of the Maastricht Treaty. The Directive gives effect to the Framework Agreement on Parental Leave agreed by representatives of employers and employees at EU level in December 1995. The member states were required to make this law by 3 June 1998. Ireland failed to implement the Directive within this time period. The Parental Leave Act, 1998, which implements the Parental Leave Directive, came into force on 3 December 1998 and provides an individual entitlement to both parents to up to 14 weeks unpaid leave from work to take care of young children. The leave was to be taken before the child reaches five years of age, except in exceptional circumstances in the case of an adopted child. Under the Act, the entitlement was restricted to parents of children born or adopted on or after the 3 June 1996. The European Commission issued a Reasoned Opinion dated 3 April 2000 to the effect that Ireland by restricting the right to parental leave to employees with children born or adopted on or after 3 June 1996 failed to fulfil its obligations under the Framework Agreement on Parental Leave. On 20 July 2000, there was an extension of the grounds by way of regulation to the Parental Leave Act 1998 by which certain categories of parents may be entitled to parental leave.

Mothers and Welfare

Social protection legislation relates to women who are participants in the labour market. But what about mothers outside the market? Women who are generally referred to as mothers in the home or homemakers, a term which suggests that those who spend some time working outside the home somehow are not homemakers. Women outside the labour market generally find they have two possible sources of finance: one is to depend on a male breadwinner for support, and the other is to depend on the state. Most women generally access financial resources from the state due to their status as mothers. Looking first at pregnant women, it is clear that what payments are available to women during the maternity period have become eroded over the decades. Cousins, in an account of the historical development of maternity rights in Ireland, indicates:

> Developments in the 1980s and 1990s have seen maternity protection being much more closely linked to participation in the paid labour force and the abolition of both maternity

grants and allowances for women who are not in employment (1995: 114–115).

Unfortunately, the many active groups in Ireland which have organised around childbirth issues — the Association for the Improvement of Maternity Services (AIMS), the Irish Association for the Improvement of Maternity Services (IAIMS), the La Leche League (LLL), and Cuidiú — have not addressed this vital issue. They have tended to concentrate on direct medical and support services for women during the maternity period.

Maternity Payments

Cousins (1992, 1995) distinguishes between two different types of maternity payments. The first are once-off cash payments, paid to women around the time of childbirth and intended to assist with the additional financial costs associated with childbirth. This includes the exceptional needs payments (ENPs), which are part of the supplementary welfare allowance scheme. The second type of payments are those designed to replace a woman's income while she is absent from the paid labour market on a temporary basis due to childbirth. There is a third type of payment which is relevant to maternity: that is, child benefit, a universal payment which exists outside of these maternity-related payments.

Looking initially at the maternity-related payments, what becomes apparent is that their real value has become eroded over the years and now the only women entitled to any direct maternity payments (apart from the €10.16 means-tested maternity grant) are those in employment (Table 11.1). These payments are now examined in detail.

Table 11.1: Chronological Development of Maternity Payments in Ireland since 1911

Year	Cash Grant (Social Insurance)	Cash Grant (Means Tested)	Maternity Payment (General Scheme) for Insured Mothers	Maternity Payment (Employment Scheme) for Insured Mothers
1911	Introduced under the 1911 National Insurance Act €1.90			
1920	Increased to €2.54 and payable on insurance record of either/both husband and wife.			
1952	Changed to maternity grant		Social Welfare Act, maternity allowance which was for six weeks before and six weeks after childbirth introduced	Social Welfare Act, maternity allowance which was for six weeks before and six weeks after childbirth introduced
1953		Introduced under the 1953 Health Act.		
1965	Increased to €5.08			
1970		Increased to €10.16		

Year	Cash Grant (Social Insurance)	Cash Grant (Means Tested)	Maternity Payment (General Scheme) for Insured Mothers	Maternity Payment (Employment Scheme) for Insured Mothers
1973			Pay-related addition was introduced	
1974	Increased to €10.16			
1981				Social Welfare (amendment) Act — 14 weeks at a rate of 80 per cent of previous earnings with a minimum of €6.03 per week
1983	Abolished	Renamed as maternity grant		
1984				Rate was reduced to 70 per cent
1987			Contribution conditions became more onerous	Contribution conditions became more onerous
1988			Pay-related benefit abolished	

Year	Cash Grant (Social Insurance)	Cash Grant (Means Tested)	Maternity Payment (General Scheme) for Insured Mothers	Maternity Payment (Employment Scheme) for Insured Mothers
1991			1991 Social Welfare Act maternity allowance was abolished	Worker Protection (Regular Part-time Employees) Act extended to include part-time workers earning over €31.74 per week
1994				Maternity (Protection of Employment) Act Health and Safety payment
1995				Adoption payment
2001				The Maternity Protection Act, 1994 (Extension of Periods of Leave) Order 2001 and the Adoptive Leave Act, 1995 (Extension of Periods of Leave) Order 2001

Source: Compiled by author from annual reports of the Department of Health and the Department of Social Welfare.

Cash Grants — Once-off Payments

The present maternity grant available from the Department of Health is a once-off means-tested payment of €10.16. This originated under the 1952 Social Welfare Act. Up until then, maternity payments were related to social insurance contributions of the mother or father. When introduced 50 years ago, the amount was the equivalent of €5.08 (worth €101.40 at 2001 prices) and is now double that figure, at €10.16, as it has been since 1970 (worth €66.99 at 2001 prices). Statistics on recent trends in the number of claims of this payment demonstrate that the number of women receiving the grant has decreased steadily over the last two decades from 8,585 recipients (11.84 per cent of births) in 1979 to 4,500 in 1999 (8.4 per cent of all births). Hence, there has been an overall saving to the state.

Cousins (1993) outlines the historical evolution of this payment and what becomes apparent from his analysis is that the grant has been consistently eroded since its introduction in 1952. This is all the worse because it is a means-tested grant that goes to poor mothers. In real terms, what can the new mother buy with this €10.16? On average a packet of disposable nappies cost between €10 and €15. This gives some indication of the value of this grant in 1998 terms. It is not surprising, therefore, that only 4,500 women in 2000, or 8.3 per cent of all women who gave birth, claimed the maternity grant. Since 1992 this means-tested payment of €10.16 is the only maternity-related payment (except for child benefit) available to all women who are not in employment on a low income.

Table 11.2: Department of Health Maternity Grant

Year	Number of Recipients	Cost (€)	Number of Births	Recipients of Grant as a % of Total Births
1979	8,585	87,205.61	72,539	11.84
1980	8,313	84,442.66	74,064	11.23
1981	7,831	79,546.55	72,158	10.85
1982	7,672	77,931.44	70,843	10.83
1984	6,108	62,044.48	64,062	9.54
1985	5,518	56,051.32	62,388	8.84
1986	5,984	60,784.90	61,620	9.71
1987	5,085	51,652.95	58,433	8.70
1988	3,963	40,255.78	54,600	7.23
1989	3,963	40,255.78	52,018	7.67
1990	3,490	35,451.09	53,044	6.60
1991	3,649	37,066.19	52,718	6.92
1992	3,544	35,999.61	51,089	6.93
1993	3,735	37,939.77	49,461	7.55
1994	3,704	37,624.88	47,928	7.72
1995	3,101	31,499.66	48,530	6.38
1997	4,250	43,171.09	52,775	8.05
1998	4,250	43,171.09	53,551	8.0
1999	4,500	45,710.57	53,354	8.4
2000*	4,500	45,710.57	54,239	8.3

Source: Compiled by author from Department of Health Statistics for 1979–2000. * Estimate

Maternity Allowance

Insurance-related maternity payments were introduced in 1911 with the National Insurance Act of that year, which legislated for the introduction of a payment called "maternity benefit", at a rate of €1.90 (worth €116.71 at 2001 prices), raised in 1920 to €2.54

(worth €76.97 at 2001 prices). The grant was payable either on the husband's or wife's insurance record and the contribution requirements were easy to satisfy. This payment was renamed "maternity grant" under the 1952 Health Act and was increased to €5.08 in 1965 (worth €66.79 at 2001 prices). This payment was abolished in 1983. This meant that the only once-off payment for women at the time of childbirth is the Department of Health €10.16 means-tested maternity grant discussed above. Table 11.3 presents data which demonstrates the numbers of grants received. In 1981, for example, there were over 50,000 grants paid and over 70,000 births. These figures do not give a true picture of the proportion of grants associated with each birth, as it is possible that one birth represents two grants in some cases, while for other births neither parent was entitled to a grant. However, it does show that the numbers of grants paid was sizeable.

Table 11.3: Total Number of Maternity Grants in Ireland

Year	Total Number of Births	Maternity Grant (man's insurance)	Maternity Grant (woman's insurance)	Total Maternity Grants
1976	67,718	30,950	17,140	48,090
1977	68,892	30,006	17,298	47,304
1978	70,299	30,104	17,059	47,163
1979	72,539	27,349	15,859	43,208
1980	74,064	27,282	17,617	44,898
1981	72,158	27,798	22,357	50,155
1982	70,843	24,149	14,909	39,055

Source: Compiled by author from Department of Social Welfare annual reports for selected years.

In 1953, a contributory "maternity allowance" was introduced under the 1952 Social Welfare Act. This was an allowance payable for six weeks before and six weeks after confinement to an insured woman who met the contribution conditions "to relieve her of the necessity of working immediately before and after the confinement" (Farley, 1964: 100). In the case of confinement being earlier than expected, the allowance was still only paid until six weeks after the confinement. It was payable on the woman's insurance only. A married woman had to have at least 26 contributions paid after her marriage before she could qualify. In October 1973, the rule which disqualified women on marriage from receiving short-term social welfare benefits until a further 26 contributions had been made was removed. Women who were outside the labour market could claim this payment as it was based on past contributions and not on current employment status.

The Social Welfare (pay-related benefit) Act 1973 provided for the introduction of a pay-related benefit scheme, which was an earnings-related supplement to the flat rate maternity allowance. It was introduced with effect from April 1974. There was a new scheme introduced in 1981 in line with the Maternity Protection of Employment Act which legislated for maternity leave. The 1986 Social Welfare Act legislated for the rationalisation of the maternity scheme for women in employment. Pay-related and flat rate elements were amalgamated and accounted for under the "maternity allowance" heading.

Table 11.4: Numbers of Awards of Maternity Protection Payments, 1970-2000

Year	Adoptive Benefit (1)	Health and Safety Benefit (2)	Maternity Benefit (3)	Employment Benefit (4)	General Scheme (5)	Total of (4) and (5)
1970	—	—	—	n/a	n/a	8,371
1971	—	—	—	n/a	n/a	9,159
1972	—	—	—	n/a	n/a	10,051
1973	—	—	—	n/a	n/a	11,091
1974	—	—	—	n/a	n/a	10,829
1975	—	—	—	n/a	n/a	15,589
1976	—	—	—	n/a	n/a	17,197
1977	—	—	—	n/a	n/a	17,189
1978	—	—	—	n/a	n/a	17,299

Year	Adoptive Benefit (1)	Health and Safety Benefit (2)	Maternity Benefit (3)	Employment Benefit (4)	General Scheme (5)	Total of (4) and (5)
1979	—	—	—	n/a	n/a	16,867
1980	—	—	—	n/a	n/a	18,489
1981	—	—	20,056	4,604	15,452	20,056
1982	—	—	23,167	9,227	10,673	19,900
1983	—	—	n/a	4,866	5,455	10,321
1984	—	—	21,525	9,317	4,022	13,339
1985	—	—	20,746	10,727	8,919	19,646
1986	—	—	20,916	11,020	790	11,810
1987	—	—	21,895	11,065	8,358	19,423
1988	—	—	19,149	2,900	805	3,705
1989	—	—	14,569	3,286	680	3,966
1990	—	—	15,529	3,900	756	4,656
1991*	—	—	16,357	4,077	670	4,747
1992	—	—	14,876	3,411	0	—
1993	—	—	15,553	3,651	0	—
1994	—	5	14,378	—	0	—
1995	52	70	15,664	—	0	—
1996	42	79	17,628			
1997	64	123	19,796			
1998	88	93	22,384	—	0	—
1999	110	125	23,851			
2000	105	96	24,848			

Source: Compiled by author from Department of Social Welfare statistics for years 1970–2000

Adoptive Benefit introduced 19 April 1995

Health and Safety Benefit introduced 19 October 1994

Maternity Benefit introduced 16 April 981

* Extended to include part-time workers earning over £25 per week.

— denotes not applicable

n/a denotes statistics not available

Table 11.5: Total Number of Recipients of Scheme for Women in Employment and General Scheme

Year	Total of (2) and (5) (1)	Number of Recipients of Scheme for Women in Employment (2)**	Number of Pay-related Payments (3)	Average weekly payment (€) (4)	Number of Recipients of General Scheme (5)*	Number of Pay-related Payments (6)	Average Weekly Payment (€) (7)
1970	8,371	n/a	n/a	n/a	n/a	n/a	n/a
1971	9,159	n/a	n/a	n/a	n/a	n/a	n/a
1972	10,051	n/a	n/a	n/a	n/a	n/a	n/a
1973	11,091	n/a	n/a	n/a	n/a	n/a	n/a
1974	10,829	n/a	n/a	n/a	n/a	n/a	n/a
1975	15,589	n/a	n/a	n/a	n/a	n/a	n/a
1976	17,197	n/a	n/a	n/a	n/a	n/a	n/a
1977	17,189	n/a	n/a	n/a	n/a	n/a	n/a
1978	17,299	n/a	n/a	n/a	n/a	n/a	n/a
1979	16,867	n/a	n/a	n/a	n/a	n/a	18.97
1980	18,489	n/a	n/a	n/a	n/a	n/a	26.17
1981	20,056	4,604	1,795	39.41	15,452	1,535	17.50
1982	19,900	9,227	2,442	49.28	10,673	1,150	20.16

Year	Total of (2) and (5) (1)	Number of Recipients of Scheme for Women in Employment (2)**	Number of Pay-related Payments (3)	Average weekly payment (€) (4)	Number of Recipients of General Scheme (5)*	Number of Pay-related Payments (6)	Average Weekly Payment (€) (7)
1983†	10,321	4,866	1,830	55.68	5,455	1,191	20.44
1984‡	18,670	9,317	7,547	22.49	9,353	4,022	16.07
1985	19,646	10,727	2,888	61.76	8,919	781	13.54
1986	19,881	11,020	n/a	n/a	8,861	790	16.05
1987	19,423	11,065	n/a	n/a	8,358	523	18.97
1988	3,705	2,900	n/a	n/a	805	–	–
1989	3,966	3,286	n/a	n/a	680	–	–
1990	4,656	3,900	n/a	n/a	756	–	–
1991	4,747	4,077	–	–	670	–	–
1992	3,411	3,411	–	–	–	–	–
1993	3,651	3,651	–	–	–	–	–

Source: Compiled by author from Department of Social Welfare statistics for years 1970–1993

* Introduced 1952; pay-related payment introduced 1974; scheme discontinued from 6 April 1992.

** Introduced 1952

† January to 30 June 1983; ‡ July 1983 to 30 June 1984

The "maternity allowance" scheme continued to apply to women who did not qualify for maternity leave under the Maternity Protection of Employees Act, 1981. However, in 1988, eligibility criteria became more onerous. From April 1988, new claims under the general maternity allowance scheme were required to have 13 weeks' paid contributions during the governing contribution year to ensure that women had recently been at work. This was an obvious policy departure, which militated against women outside the labour market and led to a huge reduction in the numbers eligible for maternity payments. Entitlement to pay-related benefit was abolished for all new claims to general maternity allowance in 1988 and from 4 April 1988, three "waiting days" were introduced for women transferring to disability benefit from maternity allowance.

Maternity Benefit

In 1981, a "maternity benefit" for women in employment was introduced under the 1981 Social Welfare Amendment Act. This was a new pay-related maternity allowance scheme and applied to women covered by the provisions of the 1981 Maternity Protection of Employees Act. The allowance was paid for 14 weeks, initially at a rate of 80 per cent of earnings reckonable for pay. This was later reduced to 75 per cent and then 70 per cent. For low earners, there is a minimum weekly payment based on average earnings of female workers in employment insurable for pay-related benefit purposes. In 1991, under the Worker Protection (Part-Time Regulations) Act, maternity benefit was extended to include part-time workers earning over €31.74 per week. In the same year, under the Social Welfare Act, the maternity allowance for those outside the labour market was abolished. Therefore, since 1991, the only payment available to women outside paid employment is the €10.16 means-tested maternity grant.

On 19 October 1994, under the Maternity Protection (Health and Safety) Act, a Health and Safety payment was introduced. It is a maternity-related social insurance payment for women whose employment is interrupted because of risk to health and/or safety related to pregnancy and/or breastfeeding and who qualify for health and safety leave. On 19 April 1995, Adoptive Benefit was introduced, being a social insurance benefit payable up to 10 weeks in cases of persons who qualify for statutory adoptive leave under the Adoptive Leave Act (No 2 of 1995); qualifying contributions and rates of payment are similar to maternity benefit. This was extended in 2001 to coincide with the extension of adoptive leave to 14 weeks.

Exceptional Needs Payments (ENPs)

Exceptional needs payments are payments made by Health Boards under the Supplementary Welfare Allowance Scheme. Under the Social Welfare (Consolidation) Act 1993, the Supplementary Welfare Allowance (SWA) scheme is administered by the Health Boards subject to the general direction and control of the Minister for Social Welfare. Section 181 of the Act provides that:

> A Health Board may, in any case where it considers it reasonable, having regard to all the circumstances of the case, so to do, determine that supplementary allowance shall be paid to a person by way of a single payment to meet an exceptional need.

This Act does not confer a statutory right or entitlement to Exceptional Needs Payments. They are discretionary payments and are concerned with once-off, exceptional circumstances. Because these payments are discretionary and thus are open to the charge of inconsistency, guidelines are laid out which state:

> In the interests of equity, where an identified need for a specific purpose is recognised by a Health Board and the applicant does not have the ability to meet it, a standard minimum ENP should be made, for example, clothing needs on admission to hospital, assistance towards the purchase of a pram, assistance on discharge from prison after a lengthy period of time (Department of Social Welfare information leaflet, 1995: 2).

The 1995 Guidelines state:

> Every decision should be based on careful consideration of all
> the circumstances of that individual case, taking account of:
> the nature and extent of the need; the availability of an alter-
> native source (other than charitable organisations) to meet, or
> partially meet, the need, for example, entitlements from other
> State agencies; the resources of the household (1995: 5).

It further indicates that when deciding a claim, the Health Board
may need to consider, in addition to the personal circumstances of
the applicant and their family, age, health, family composition,
length of time on social welfare or health board payments, pros-
pects of obtaining work, domestic or social problems. Therefore,
the pregnant woman who is in financial need and may require
assistance to buy maternity clothes has to approach the community welfare officer in her area, verify her pregnancy status and
put forward her case. Figures for 2000 indicate that a woman is
usually given about €77 towards the purchase of maternity
clothes. This is a paltry sum by today's standards. However, the
community welfare officers state that it is appropriate given that
women generally know that they are pregnant and have a few
months to budget before they may need maternity clothes. As the
woman's pregnancy draws to a close and her hospital stay draws
nearer, she may once again approach the community welfare officer for assistance towards items she may need during her hospital
stay. Looking at statistics for the ERHA indicates that in 2000
1,823 payments were made to women in the ERHA in relation to
confinement. This must be viewed in the context of over 15,000
women giving birth there in that year. The total cost was
€139,790.96 (Table 11.6).

Table 11.6: Number of Exceptional Needs Payments (ENPs) for 1999 and 2000 in the ERHA

	1999	2000
Prams and buggies		
Payments	4,419	4,466
Amount	€579,758.37	€594,025.37
Average	(€131)	(€133)
Cots		
Payments	3,158	3,399
Amount	€404,184.57	€441,107.68
Average	(€128)	(€130)
Confinement		
Payments	1,367	1,823
Amount	€99,854.74	€139,790.96
Average	(€73)	(€77)

Source: Figures provided by ISTS Department, ERHA.

When women attend a maternity unit for ante-natal care, they are given a list of items which they are required to bring to the hospital with them when they are in labour. The list issued by the Rotunda for the year 2000/2001 is presented below, followed by an approximate total costing calculated in Dunnes Stores, one of the least expensive department stores in Ireland.

Maternity patients:

- Two night dresses

- Dressing gown

- Slippers

- Personal toilet requisites including: panties, bra, sanitary towels.

Post-delivery:

- Two night dresses

- Two pairs of panties

- One bra.

For baby:

- Two babygrows/gowns

- Two vests

- Two cardigans

- Two towels

- Disposable nappies

- Baby cream

- Cotton wool

- Baby bath lotion.

Even with this conservative estimated costing, the Rotunda's list at approximately €146 is hardly compatible with the ERHA's average payment of €77.

This has to be viewed in the context of the emotions and expectations of a woman about to give birth to a new baby, who is going in to a hospital ward, where she will be on public view, will be with other women with whom she will undoubtedly compare herself. The woman who has a beautiful new baby who she wants to dress in the best possible clothes is definitely constrained by the Health Board guidelines. Hence, the reality of commodification for the new mother as carer, earner and lifegiver becomes painfully evident.

Once the baby is born, the Health Board, under the ENP Scheme, gives the woman a payment of €130 towards a pram or buggy. The average price of a buggy for a newborn baby is €200–€250. In 2000, there were 4,466 payments made in respect of buggies at an overall cost of €594,025.37. The average payment was €133. In addition, 3,399 cots were paid for at a cost of €441,107.68.

Participation in the normal life of society should be an attainable goal for all Irish women at all stages of the lifecycle and women should not be disadvantaged because of their "maternity status". Women turning to the Health Board to meet their most basic requirements in terms of maternity items must turn to a system of discretionary payments. Such women are denied the same standards as women who have higher incomes. While discretionary payments, such as exceptional needs payments, differentiate between women according to need, there is another very important payment to which all Irish mothers are entitled and this is child benefit.

Child Benefit

All women in Ireland who fulfil residency requirements are entitled to child benefit. It is a universal payment and one that is controversial: on the one hand, it has been criticised for not targeting those in most need; on the other hand, it has been welcomed by those who recognise it as the only payment which is paid directly to the mother regardless of her means or marital status. It is also viewed as a payment which acknowledges women's mothering role, and as a payment to which children are entitled in their own right and so acknowledges them as citizens. The distribution of income within households has not been analysed in any great depth in Ireland, with the exception of Rottman's 1994 study, which has been criticised for the sample size and methodology (Coakley, 1997). Rottman draws on the work of Jan Pahl (1990) who analyses the distribution of income within households, using the black box as an analogy to describe the household. Money goes in one side as income and comes out the other side as expenditure, but how that money is distributed within the household is not clear.

Table 11.7: Chronological Development of Child Benefit in Ireland

Year	Development
1943	Children's allowance bill
1944	Non-contributory To all families Third and subsequent child No means test Half crown a week
1952	Increase in payment Extension to second child Monthly rather than weekly
1963	Payments increased and extended to first child.
1974	Mothers became the direct beneficiaries of child benefit.
1973	Extended to children in full-time education up to age 18.
1996	Extended to children in full-time education up to age 19.

Source: Table compiled by author.

In 1952, when the children's allowance payment was changed from a weekly to a monthly payment, the then Minister for Social Welfare stated "beneficiaries should be given the opportunity of devoting allowances to . . . long-term expenditure such as the purchase of clothes and footwear than to maintenance from day to day". To apply this to today's mother, what can be bought? Kiely (2002) argues that "while the Government does not have a clearly stated family income support policy the trend since the mid-1990s has been to increase child benefit". He indicates that in 2001 child benefit was increased by 34 per cent. This is in keeping with the Government target to substantially increase child benefit over the three-year period beginning in 2000. These are in line with the National Children's Strategy target of reducing child poverty.

CONCLUSION

In conclusion, this chapter draws attention to the extent to which Irish women, throughout the maternity period, are commodified. Those with purchasing power have choice and a certain amount of autonomy, while those without such purchasing power are limited in the choices they have to make. What emerges is a picture of women having to turn to a multiplicity of sources to meet their needs as pregnant women and new mothers. Many women are deprived of choice, control, autonomy and dignity, while at the same time allocated insufficient time in which to give birth, recover, nurse and return to the labour market.

Chapter Twelve

WOMEN AS EARNERS, CARERS AND LIFEGIVERS

It is now time to return to the conceptual framework of Chapter Two, which presented women's journey through the maternity period in the context of language, time, fear, fragmentation, choice, control, dignity, cost, power, place, health and safety. In conclusion, this chapter now draws together all three dimensions of women's life with reference to these concepts, keeping in mind the social and medical models of childbirth also presented in Chapter Two. However, first it is necessary to refer to an important development in Ireland regarding the registration of births. This exemplifies the complexity for women in Ireland in officially recording the reality of their roles in society.

In September 1997, a leaflet was published by the General Register Office to assist parents in registering the birth of their child. The Registration of Births Act 1996 applies to all births registered on or after the 1 October 1997. It provides for the registration of additional information to that which was previously recorded. This is the surname of the child, the mother's address and occupation and any former surnames of the father. Up until this Act, there was no place on the registration form for the mother to record her occupation and also, in the case of married mothers, the child was automatically given the father's surname.

Significantly, for births registered after 1 October 1997, a surname can be assigned to the child, which was not always the case. The surname can be that of the father, the mother, or both. Interestingly, the guidelines refer specifically to the parent who is not employed outside the home and says that:

> . . . where a parent is currently not employed outside the home the last previously held occupation should be given. The term unemployed should not be entered on the Birth Register.

Thus, we have a ludicrous situation where a parent who is full-time in the home must deny this status and revert back to a former status, which is no longer relevant. Thus, many women in Ireland are required by law to deny their status as full-time carers. Not only is the group rendered as invisible but their true positions are also devalued.

LANGUAGE

The services women use during the maternity period are shrouded in language. In Ireland, the woman who is pregnant is said to be "expecting". What can this woman expect from the Irish social services? What she can expect in terms of social policy is related to her status in the labour force. The language, definitions, measurements used by the Labour Force Surveys and the Live Register fail to name or categorise mothers. What can women expect? The woman outside the labour market can expect to depend on a male breadwinner or the discretionary exceptional needs payments or a universal benefit called "child benefit". Where is motherhood valued in this language? The woman is named as a "patient" by the health services and a "claimant" by the welfare services. The woman is granted leave from employment to give birth and the woman in the home is not even mentioned. The woman in the labour force can claim health and safety leave, but whose health and whose safety is at issue here? In this cloud of language, motherhood remains a mystery.

TIME

Time is vital. Time to gestate, time to deliver. Time to bond, time to attach, time to care, time to recover. For mothers in the home full-time, it is assumed that they have time. For mothers in the paid labour market, time is allocated. This is named "maternity leave" but in effect it is time allowed out of the labour market. Interestingly, in Ireland the six weeks postpartum is marked by a post-natal visit which marks the end of entitlement to free health care under the Maternity and Infant Care Scheme. A mother and six-week-old baby are then expected to no longer need free medical services. It is time for services to let go, and for the majority of mothers and their children to depend on their own resources.

Glendinning and Millar (1992) refer to poverty of time. Outside the labour market, time is generally uncosted and in the postpartum period women soon learn that childcare involves time. Looking at advice presented in the *Baby Care Guide* (1995) dispensed by public health nurses to pregnant women:

> You don't yet realise that it is normal for a baby to take over a mother's life during the early weeks . . . you have yet to accept that all babies cry at times — the average total is two hours a day in the first month or so, according to research (1995: 4).

This patronising booklet also outlines the need for the mother to cater for the needs of the child's father and siblings as "there is a risk that your partner may feel 'left out' and rejected . . . older children often feel unloved and displaced by a new brother or sister" (1995: 5). Time is an issue for nursing mothers. Women in the labour force are entitled to a maximum of 14 weeks' paid postnatal leave but are encouraged to breastfeed for a minimum of four months (Department of Health, 1994d). How can these conflicting time scales be reconciled when only a minute number of workplace crèches exist in Ireland?

FEAR

For the woman experiencing the maternity period, there is always the shadow of fear. For some there is the fear of childbirth. For others there is the fear of having to stay at home alone with a new baby with little financial or social support. For others there is the fear of returning to employment, fear of leaving the child, of not finding and being able to afford adequate child care. For some there is the fear of facing the community welfare officer for financial support. For many there is the fear of obstetric practices and hospitalisation for themselves or their children.

FRAGMENTATION

In Chapter Seven, a model of welfare pluralism was introduced which categorises four different sectors: the statutory sector, the voluntary sector, the private and the informal. Looking at welfare services for women during the maternity period, mothers are fragmented into two groups: those with purchasing power and those without. To where does the latter group turn? They must turn to the community welfare service or to the informal sector, friends, sisters or relations who may have clothes to share. Others will out of necessity turn to the voluntary sector and groups such as St Vincent de Paul. On the other hand, those with purchasing power can go to stores like Mothercare which target pregnant women with their expensive advertising campaigns.

CHOICE

New mothers in Ireland find themselves faced with very limited choices. For women who are returning to the labour market, they have the choice to take an extra eight weeks' unpaid leave. This might be a choice for some but not for others, and either way has implications for breastfeeding practices. For many women, the choice to stay longer with the child, to care for it during the early ages of its life, does not exist. Parallel to this is the virtual absence of good quality, affordable childcare. In this sphere in Ireland, women have little choice. Choice in terms of job-sharing, flexitime and flexi-place does not exist for most women in Ireland.

CONTROL

Women when pregnant can feel very much out of control; their lives can seem to be subsumed by the responsibility for the child they are carrying. They can feel caught up in a series of hospital appointments, examinations and dates. This lack of control is experienced by women who feel forced to return to work, forced to discontinue breastfeeding because they have no control over working conditions, environment and times of work, no access to flexible working times and arrangements.

DIGNITY

Issues of choice and dignity are important here. Purchasing power dictates choice. Some women are robbed of their dignity. When, for example, it comes to needing special underwear, dignity should be assured. In Ireland, a pregnant woman may find herself in a situation where she is in a health board office with a community welfare officer, a stranger who may not necessarily be sensitive or caring where she has to discuss her most intimate needs, verify her pregnancy status and ask for financial assistance to purchase the most basic necessities. By the end of the nine months, the pregnant woman will have become a totally different shape and weight. At a most basic level, women need new clothes while they are pregnant — maternity clothes, not necessarily "bigger" clothes which is the simplistic understanding often put forward. Also, on a very practical basis, pregnant women tend to need to change their clothes more frequently for reasons of personal hygiene; yet they may find they are too exhausted to wash their clothes as frequently as they may wish. Having to point this out to a community welfare officer does little for one's dignity. Similarly, applying for a €10.16 maternity grant does not leave the applicant with much pride and self-esteem. For the lactating mother, returning to work and trying to hide the fact that one's breasts are engorged, sore and leaking does not leave one feeling very dignified.

COST

Pregnancy and childbirth involve risk. They take energy and time. They take a woman's time, but a woman's time in society has traditionally been uncounted and uncosted. This is true also for the time spent gestating and lactating as well as caring. It involves physical, emotional and psychological expenditure. Having children costs money. The infant receiving care has needs, which it is generally assumed the mother will meet. These needs are both emotional — love, nurturing, bonding — and physical — clothes, shelter and food. Symonds and Hunt refer to having a baby as a form of economic suicide. They refer to "the contradiction between the relatively high ideological status given to motherhood and the correspondingly low economic status which it confers" (1996: 113).

POWER

Mothers often describe childbirth as empowering. Others describe it in terms of abuse, violation and powerlessness. The woman without financial power is dependent on her partner or the state. Some partners are generous. Others are not. Women availing of the services of the community welfare officer also refer to their powerlessness and this is matched by their powerlessness in today's consumerist society, when they realise that, in shopping for essential maternity and baby items, they have no purchasing power. And of course, the medicalisation of childbirth itself has removed the power of women over their own bodies.

PLACE

The pregnant woman is concerned with places — places in which to give birth, whether home or hospital, private or public wards. The new mother is concerned with places — places to go to get social support, to meet other mothers, to learn how to parent. The woman returning to the workplace is concerned with childcare places, distance to work from the place where the child is being cared for and the lack of availability of workplace nurseries. For the fortunate mother who has been able to make a satisfactory childcare arrangement for her child, who has a loving supportive spouse and a reasonable job, home although much busier with a new baby can be a haven of solace and renewal after a hectic day at her job.

HEALTH

The Irish health services attempt to cater for the basic health needs of mother and infant, employing a medical model of health. Policies which dictate that a woman must leave her child and return to the workforce within an allocated time rather than according to individual needs of mother and baby cannot guarantee good physical, psychological and emotional health. Such policies are not synonymous with good nutrition for the baby and the provision of rest and relaxation for the mother.

SAFETY

A safe home to which the mother can return with her infant after birth is essential for the health and safety of both. Support within this home is also essential. Some women do not have such a secure physical and social environment. Traveller women often have to mother in sub-standard conditions, as do women from lower socio-economic groups. Social support is something that cannot be taken for granted by either the mother who has a partner or the lone mother. Some women miss out on an emotionally warm and safe home for themselves and their children. Irish women have to take at least four weeks' maternity leave from paid employment prior to the expected date of delivery. Many women concerned with the inadequacy of maternity leave in the postpartum period lie about their expected date of delivery in order to work until a later date in the pregnancy. This has repercussions for the safety of both the baby and the mother.

BIBLIOGRAPHY

Ainsworth S.M.D. (1991) "Attachments and other Affectional Bonds Across the Life Cycle", in Parkes, C.M., Stevenson-Hinde, J. and Marris, P. (eds.), *Attachment Across the Lifecycle*, pp. 33–51, Routledge, London and New York.

Aldous, J. et al. (1999) *Refugee Health in London: Key Issues for Public Health*, Health of Londoners Project, East London and the City Health Authority.

Alexander, J. and Levy, V. (1990) *Post-natal Care: A Research Based Approach*, Macmillan, Basingstoke.

Alexander J., Levy, V. and Roch, S. (eds.) (1990) *Ante-natal Care: A Research Based Approach*, Macmillan, Basingstoke.

Alexander J., Levy, V. and Roch, S. (eds.) (1995) *Aspects of Midwifery Practice: A Research Based Approach*, Macmillan, London.

Allal, P., Kell, T., Bryman, A. and Blylheway, B. (1987) *Women and the Life Cycle, Transitions and Turning Points*, St. Martin's Press, New York.

An Bord Altranais (1994) *The Future of Nurse Education and Training in Ireland*, An Bord Altranais, Dublin.

Archer, J. (1976) "Biological Explanations of Psychological Sex Differences", in Lloyd, B. and Archer, J. (eds.), *Exploring Sex Differences*, Academic Press, London.

Arditti, R. (1984) *Test-Tube Women: What Future for Motherhood?* Pandora Press, London.

Athey, J. and Ahearn, F. (1991) "The Mental Health of Refugee Children: An Overview", in Ahearn, F. and Athey, J. (eds.), *Refugee Children: Theory, Research and Services*, Johns Hopkins University, Baltimore and London.

Atkinson, C.W. (1991) *The Oldest Vocation: Christian Motherhood in the Middle Ages*, Cornell University, New York.

Audit Commission (1998) *First Class Delivery: A National Survey of Women's Views of Maternity Care,* Audit Commission for Local Authorities/National Perinatal Epidemiology Unit, London.

Badinter, E. (1981) *The Myth of Motherhood: An Historical View of the Maternal Instinct,* Souvenir Press, London.

Balaskas, A.J. (1979) *New Life: The Book of Exercises for Childbirth,* Anchor Press, London.

Ball, J.A. (1989) "Postnatal Care and Adjustment to Motherhood", in Robinson, S. and Thomson, A.M. (eds.), *Midwives, Research and Childbirth,* Vol. 1, Chapman and Hall, London.

Ball, J.A. (1994) *Reactions to Motherhood: The Role of Post-natal Care,* (2nd edition), Books for Midwives, Hull.

Banks, O. (1986) *Faces of Feminism: A Study of Feminism as a Social Movement,* Martin Robertson, Oxford.

Barnes, C. (1997) "A Legacy of Oppression: A History of Disability in Western Culture" in Barton, L. and Oliver, M. (eds.), *Disability Studies, Past, Present and Future,* The Disability Press, Leeds, pp. 3–24.

Barrett, M. (1980) *Women's Oppression Today: The Marxist/Feminist Encounter,* Verso, London.

Barrett, M. and McIntosh, M. (1991) *The Anti-Social Family,* Verso, London.

Barrington, R. (1987) *Health, Medicine and Politics in Ireland, 1900–1970,* Institute of Public Administration, Dublin.

Barry, U. (1992) "Movement Change and Reaction: The Struggle over Reproductive Rights in Ireland" in Smyth A. (ed.), *The Abortion Papers,* Attic Press, Dublin.

Barry, J., Herity, B. and Solan, J. (1989) *The Travellers' Health Status Study: Vital Statistics of Travelling People,* Dublin, Health Research Board.

Beale, J. (1986) *Women in Ireland: Voices of Change,* Macmillan, London.

Beech, B. and Robinson, J. (1994) *Ultrasound? Unsound,* Association for Improvements in the Maternity Services, London.

Begley, C.M. (1987) "Episiotomy: A Change in Midwives Practice", *Irish Nursing Forum and Health Studies,* Nov/Dec.

Begley, C.M. (1990) "A Comparison of 'Active' and 'Physiological' Management of the Third Stage of Labour", *Midwifery,* 6, pp. 8–17.

Begley, C.M. (1991) "Post-partum Haemorrhage: Who is at Risk? *Midwives Chronicle*, 104, pp. 102–106.

Begley, C.M. (1997) *Midwives in the Making: A Longitudinal Study of the Experiences of Student Midwives during their Two Year Training in Ireland*, unpublished PhD thesis, Dublin University, Trinity College, Dublin.

Begley, C.M. (1998) "Explaining Post-partum Haemorrhage: The Value of a Physiological Third Stage" in Kennedy, P. and Murphy Lawless, J. (eds.), *Returning Birth to Women: Challenging Policy and Practice*, Women's Education and Research Resource Centre, UCD, and Centre for Women's Studies, TCD.

Begum, N. (1992) "Disabled Women and the Feminist Agenda", *Feminist Review*, 40, pp. 70–84.

Begum, N. (1996) "Doctor, Doctor . . . Disabled Women's Experiences of General Practitioners", in Morris, J. (ed.), *Encounters with Strangers: Feminism and Disability — The Major Issue Confronting Feminism Today*, The Women's Press, London, pp. 168-193.

Benn, M. (1998) *Madonna and Child: Towards a New Politics of Motherhood*, Jonathan Cape, London.

Beveridge, W. (1942) *Social Insurance and Allied Services*, Cmnd. 6404, HMSO, London.

Billington, R. (1994) *The Great Umbilical: Mothers, Daughters, Mothers, the Unbreakable Bond*, Hutchinson, London.

Blomquist, H. and Soderman, P. (1991) "The Occurrence of Symptoms and the Proportion Treated in Swedish Infants and their Mothers", *Scandinavian Journal of Primary Health Care*, 9, pp. 217–223.

Borchorst, A. (1990) "Political Motherhood and Childcare Policies: A Comparative Approach to Britain and Scandinavia", in Ungerson, C. (ed.), *Gender and Caring, Work and Welfare in Britain and Scandinavia*, Harvester Wheatsheaf, London.

Bourke, M. (1997) *Working with Drug Users in General Practice*, EHB/ICGP, Dublin.

Bourne, G. (1989) *Pregnancy*, Pan Books, London.

Bowlby, J. (1951) *Maternal Care and Mental Health*, WHO, Geneva.

Bowlby, J. (1953) *Child Care and the Growth of Love*, Penguin, Harmondsworth.

Bradshaw, J. and Ditch, J. (1994) "A Comparison of the Structure and Level of Financial Support for Children in Ireland and Seventeen Other Countries", Paper for Seminar *Family Income Support in Ireland — 50 Years On*, Department of Social Welfare and European Institute of Social Security (Irish Branch), Dublin Castle, 23 September.

Bradshaw, J., Ditch, J., Holmes, H. and Whiteford, P. (1993) "A Comparative Study of Child Support in Fifteen Countries", *Journal of European Social Policy*, 3 (4), pp. 317–318.

Breen, R., Hannan, F., Rottman, D. and Whelan, C. (1990) *Understanding Contemporary Ireland: State, Class and Development in the Republic of Ireland*, Gill & Macmillan, Dublin.

Browne, N. (1986) *Against the Tide*, Gill and Macmillan, Dublin.

Bunreacht na hÉireann (Constitution of Ireland) (1937) Government Publications, Dublin.

Burke, H. (1987) *The People and the Poor Law in 19th Century Ireland*, The Women's Education Bureau, Dublin.

Burke, H. (1993) *The Royal Hospital Donnybrook: A Heritage of Caring, 1743–1993*, Royal Hospital Donnybrook/Social Science Research Centre, UCD.

Butler, S. and Woods, M. (1992) "Drugs, HIV and Ireland: Responses to Women in Dublin" in Dorn, N., Henderson, S. and South, N. (eds.), *AIDS, Women, Drugs and Social Care*, Falmer Press, London.

Byrne, A. and Leonard, M. (eds.) (1997) *Women and Irish Society: A Sociological Reader*, Beyond the Pale, Belfast.

Byrne, B., Cotter, A., Molloy, E. and Turner, M. (1998) "Should Pregnant Women be Screened for Drugs of Abuse?", *Irish Medical Journal*, Jan/Feb, Vol. 91, No. 1.

Byrne-Lynch, A. (1991) "Coping Strategies, Personal Control and Childbirth", *Irish Journal of Psychology*, Vol. 12, No. 2, pp. 145–152.

Campbell, J.C. (1995) "Addressing Battering during Pregnancy: Reducing Low Birth Weight and Ongoing Abuse", *Seminars in Perinatalogy*, Vol. 19, No. 4 (August), pp. 301–306.

Campbell, R. (1984) "Home Births in England and Wales: Perinatal Mortality According to Intended Place of Delivery", *British Medical Journal*, 289, pp. 721–724.

Campbell, R. and MacFarlane, A. (1995) *Where to be Born? The Debate and the Evidence* (2nd edition; 1st edition, 1987), Crown Publications for National Perinatal Epidemiology Unit, Oxford.

Campbell, R. and MacFarlane, A. (1990) "Recent Debate on the Place of Birth", in Garcia, J. et al. (eds.), *The Politics of Maternity Care*, Clarendon Press, Oxford.

Caplan, P. (ed.) (1987) *The Cultural Construction of Sexuality*, Routledge, London.

Carney, C. (1991) *Selectivity Issues in Irish Social Services*, Family Services Centre, University College Dublin.

Carter, P. (1995) *Feminism, Breasts and Breastfeeding*, Macmillan, London.

Central Statistics Office (1983) *Report on Vital Statistics*, Stationery Office, Dublin.

Central Statistics Office (1991), *Census of Population*, Stationery Office, Dublin.

Central Statistics Office (1995) *Labour Force Projections*, Stationery Office, Dublin.

Central Statistics Office (1996a) *Census of Population*, Stationery Office, Dublin.

Central Statistics Office (1996b) *Labour Force Survey*, Stationery Office, Dublin.

Central Statistics Office (1997), *Women in the Workforce*, Statistical Release, September, Dublin and Cork.

Central Statistics Office (2001), *Quarterly National Household Survey Households and Family Units*, 28 November, Stationery Office, Dublin.

Chalmers, A. (1993) "Effective Care in Midwifery: Research, the Professions and the Public", *Midwives Chronicle and Nursing Notes*, January, pp. 3–14.

Chalmers, B. (1997) "Changing Childbirth in Eastern Europe" in Davis-Floyd, R. and Sergeant, C. (eds.), *Childbirth: An Authoritative Knowledge, Cross-cultural Perspectives*, University of California, Berkeley.

Chamberlain, G. (1978) *British Births 1970, Vol. 2, Obstetric Care*, Heinemann. London.

Chamberlain, G. (1995) *Obstetrics by Ten Teachers* (16th edition), Arnold, London.

Chesler, P. (1990) *Sacred Bond: Motherhood under Siege, Surrogacy, Adoption and Custody*, Virago, London.

Chodorow, N. (1978) *The Reproduction of Mothering: Psychoanalysis and the Sociology of Gender*, University of California Press, Berkeley and London.

Churcher, M. (1997) "Midwifery Care for Travellers" in Karger, I. and Hunt, S. (eds.), *Challenges in Midwifery Care*, Macmillan, Basingstoke.

Citizen Traveller: National Survey, Attitudes to Travellers and Minority Groups, March 2000, Behaviour and Attitudes Ltd., Dublin.

Clarke, S., Keenan, E., Bergin, C., Lyons, F., Hopkins, S. and Mulcahy, F. (2001a) "The Changing Epidemiology of HIV Infection in Injecting Drug Users in Dublin, Ireland", *HIV Med*, October, 2 (4), pp. 236–240.

Clarke, S., Bergin, C., Butler, K.M., Horgan, M. and Sheehan, G. (2001b) "National Guidelines for the Active Management of HIV in Pregnancy, Working Party Report", *Irish Medical Journal*, May, Vol. 94, No. 5.

Coakley, A. (1997) "Gendered Citizenship: The Social Construction of Mothers in Ireland", in Byrne, A. and Leonard, M. (eds.), *Women and Irish Society: A Sociological Reader*, Beyond the Pale, Belfast, pp. 181–195.

Cochrane, A. and Clarke, J. (eds.) (1993) *Comparing Welfare States: Britain in an International Context*, Open University, Sage, London.

Cohan, A.S. (1972) *The Irish Political Elite*, Gill and Macmillan, Dublin.

Colgan, K. (1994) *If it Happens to You: Miscarriage and Stillbirth — A Human Insight, "Glen's Story"*, Karina Colgan, Dublin.

Colwill, J. (1994) "Beveridge, Women and the Welfare State", *Critical Social Policy*, Issue 41, Autumn, pp. 53–78.

Comaroff, J. (1977) "Conflicting Paradigms of Pregnancy: Managing Ambiguity in Antenatal Encounters", in Davies, A. and Horob, G. (eds.), *Medical Encounters*, Croom Helm, London.

Combat Poverty Agency (1994) *Disability, Exclusion and Poverty Papers from the National Conference Disability, Exclusion and Poverty organised by the CPA, Forum for People with Disabilities and the NRB*, Dublin.

Comhairle na nOspidéal (1976) *Development of Hospital Maternity Services — A Discussion Document*, Dublin.

Commission of the European Communities (1993) *The Europeans and the Family: Results of an Opinion Survey*, Directorate General V: Employment, Industrial Relations and Social Affairs, Brussels.

Commission of the European Communities Childcare Network (1994) *Leave Arrangements for Workers with Children, a Review of Leave Arrangements in the Member States of the European Union and Austria, Finland, Norway and Sweden*, European Commission Network on Childcare, European Commission, Equal Opportunities Unit, Brussels

Commission on the Status of Women (1972), *Report to the Minister for Finance,* Stationery Office, Dublin.

Connolly, J., Cullen, J.H. and MacDonald, D. (1981) "Breastfeeding Practice and Factors Related to Choice of Feeding Method", *Irish Medical Journal,* 74 (6), pp. 166–168.

Conroy Jackson, P. (1993) "Managing the Mothers: The Case of Ireland", in Lewis, J. (ed.), *Women and Social Policies in Europe: Work, Family and the State,* Edward Elgar, New York.

Conroy, P. (1997) "Lone Mothers: The Case of Ireland", in Lewis, J. (ed.), *Lone Mothers in European Welfare Regimes: Shifting Policy Logics,* Jessica Kingsley, London.

Conroy, P. and McDermott, M. (2001) *Extract from the Final Report of Volunteering and the Organisation,* part of a research study undertaken by Ralaheen Ltd. for Comhairle and the Irish National Committee on Volunteering in the context of the United Nations International Year of the Volunteer, Ralaheen Ltd., Dublin.

Consultative Council on General Hospital Services (1968) *Outline of the Future Hospital System,* Stationery Office, Dublin.

Coombe Women's Hospital (previously the Coombe Lying-in Hospital), *Annual Clinical Reports* 1970–2000 (30 reports).

Cooney, J. (1986) *The Crozier and the Dáil, Church and State, 1922–1986,* Mercier Press, Cork.

Corea, G. (1998) *The Mother Machine,* The Women's Press, London.

Cosslett, T. (1994) *Women Writing Childbirth, Modern Discourses of Motherhood,* Manchester University Press, Manchester.

Coulter, C. (1993) *The Hidden Tradition: Feminism, Women and Nationalism in Ireland,* Undercurrents Series, Cork University Press, Cork.

Council of European Communities (1980) Council Directive (80/155/EEC) *Concerning the mutual recognition of diplomas, certificates and other evidence of qualification in midwifery and including measures to facilitate the effective exercise of the right of establishment and freedom to provide services,* Council of European Communities, Brussels.

Cousins, M. (1992) "Pregnancy and Maternity Benefits: A Case Study of Irish Social Welfare Provision", *Administration,* Vol. 4, No. 3, pp. 220–233, Institute of Public Administration, Dublin.

Cousins, M. (1995) *Social Welfare and the Law in Ireland,* Macmillan, Dublin.

Cousins, M. (1996) *Pathways to Employment for Women Returning to Paid Work: Access to the Live Register*, Employment Equality Agency, Dublin.

Cox, G., O'Shea, M. and Geoghegan, T. (1999) "Gender Differences in Characteristics of Drug Users Presenting to Dublin Syringe Exchange", *Irish Journal of Psychological Medicine*, 16 (4) pp.131-135

Creasy, R. (1991) "Preventing Preterm Birth", *New England Journal of Medicine*, Vol. 25, No. 10, p. 727.

Creegan, M. (1967) *Unmarried Mothers An Analysis and Discussion of Interviews Conducted in an Irish Mother and Baby Home*, M.Soc.Sc. Degree (unpublished) Thesis, UCD, Dublin.

Creyghton, M. (1992) "Breast-feeding and Baraka in Northern Tunisia", in Maher, V., *The Anthropology of Breast-feeding, Natural Law or Social Construct*, Berg, Oxford.

Crow, L. (1996) "Including All of Our Lives: Renewing the Social Model of Disability" in Morris, J. (1996) (ed.), *Encounters with Strangers: Feminism and Disability — The Major Issue Confronting Feminism Today*, The Women's Press. London, pp. 206–226.

Crowley, N. (1999) "Travellers and Social Policy", in Quin, S., Kennedy, P., O'Donnell, A. and Kiely, G. (eds.), *Contemporary Irish Social Policy*, UCD Press, Dublin, pp. 243–265.

Cullen, P. (2000) *Refugees and Asylum Seekers in Ireland*, Undercurrents Series. Cork University Press, Cork.

Currell, R. (1990) "The Organisation of Midwifery Care" in Alexander, J., Levy, V. and Roch, S. (eds.), *Antenatal Care: A Research Based Approach*, Macmillan, London.

Curry, J. (1993) *The Irish Social Services*, Institute of Public Administration, Dublin.

Curtin, C., Jackson, P. and O'Connor, B. (1987) *Gender in Irish Society*, Galway University Press, Galway.

Cusimano, M. (2000) "Refugee Flows" in Cusimano, M. (ed.), *Beyond Sovereignty: Issues for a Global Agenda*, Bedford/St. Martin's Press, New York.

Dalley, G. (1988a) "Ideologies of Care: A Feminist Contribution to the Debate", *Critical Social Policy*, Issue 8, pp. 72–81.

Dalley, G. (1988b) *Ideologies of Caring*, Macmillan, Basingstoke.

Dally, A. (1982) *Inventing Motherhood, the Consequences of an Ideal*, Burnett, London.

Daly, M. (1978) *Gyn/Ecology: The Metaethics of Radical Feminism*, Beacon Press, Boston.

Daly, M. (1984) *Pure Lust: Elemental Feminist Philosophy*, Beacon Press, London.

Daly, M. (1989) *Women and Poverty*, Attic Press, Dublin.

Daly, M. (2002) "Care as a Good for Social Policy", *Journal of Social Policy*, 31, 2, pp. 251–270.

Daly, M.E. (1978) "Women, Work and Trade Unionism" in MacCurtain, M., and Ó Corrain, D. (eds.), *Women in Irish Society: The Historical Dimension*, Arlen House, Dublin, pp. 71–81.

Daly, M.E. (1995) "Women in the Irish Free State, 1922–1939: The Interaction between Economics and Ideology", *Journal of Women's History*, Vol. 6, No. 4, Vol. 7, No. 1 (Winter/Spring), pp. 99–116.

Davies, J. (1994) *Report of the Newcastle Region Home Birth Survey 1993*, North and Yorkshire Health Authority.

Davis, E. (1992) *Heart and Hands: A Midwife's Guide to Pregnancy and Birth*, Celestial Arts, Berkeley, CA.

De Vries, R. (1989) "Caregivers in Pregnancy and Childbirth", in Enkin, M. et al. (eds.), *Effective Care in Pregnancy and Childbirth*, Oxford University Press, Oxford.

Delphy, C. and Leonard, D. (1992) *Familiar Exploitation: New Analysis of Marriage in Contemporary Western Societies*, Polity Press in association with Blackwell, Cambridge.

Dempsey, A. and Mulcahy, H. (1998) *Domiciliary Midwifery and the Public Health Nursing Service*, South Eastern Health Board Waterford Community Care Area.

Department of Health (1966) *District Nursing Service: Circular issued to each Health Authority as Directed by the Minister for Health (D. O'Malley)* by P.S. O'Muireadhaigh, Secretary to the Department, Circular 27/66.

Department of Health (1981) *Health Care for Mothers and Infants: A Review of Health Care for Mothers and Infants*, Dublin.

Department of Health (1989) *Commission on Health Funding*, Dublin.

Department of Health (1993a) *Health Statistics 1993*, Stationery Office, Dublin.

Department of Health (1993b) *Perinatal Statistics, 1990*, Stationery Office, Dublin.

Department of Health (1994a) *Perinatal Statistics, 1991*, Stationery Office, Dublin.

Department of Health (1994b) *Report of the Maternity and Infant Care Scheme Review Group*, unpublished.

Department of Health (1994c) *Shaping a Healthier Future: A Strategy for Effective Healthcare in the 1990s*, Stationery Office, Dublin.

Department of Health (1994d) *A National Breastfeeding Policy for Ireland*, Stationery Office, Dublin.

Department of Health (1995) *Developing a Policy for Women's Health: A Discussion Document*, Dublin.

Department of Health (1996) *Report of the Department of Health Cervical Screening Committee*, Dublin.

Department of Health (1997a) *A Plan for Women's Health, 1997–1999*, Dublin.

Department of Health (1997b) *Report of the Maternity and Infant Care Scheme Review Group*, Department of Health, Dublin.

Department of Health and Children (2000) *AIDS Strategy 2000 — Report of the National AIDS Strategy Committee*, Dublin.

Department of Health and Children (2001) *Report of the Surveillance Sub-Committee of the National AIDS Strategy Committee on Anonymous Unlinked Antenatal HIV Screening in Ireland*, Dublin.

Department of Health and Children (2002) *Traveller Health: A National Strategy 2002–2005*, Dublin.

Department of Health, Great Britain (1993) *Changing Childbirth Part I — The Report of the Expert Maternity Group*, HMSO, London.

Department of Health, Great Britain (1999) *Guidelines for Health Workers Providing Care for Kosovan Refugees*, Unpublished.

Department of Health and Social Services (DHSS) (NI) (1994) *Delivering Choice: Midwife and General Practitioner Led Maternity Units: Report of the Northern Ireland Maternity Unit Study Group (MUSG)*, Belfast.

Department of Health and Social Services (DHSS) (NI) (1995) *Strategy for Nursing, Midwifery and Health Visiting, Action Plan for Midwives*, Belfast.

Department of Health, General Medical Services Division (1986) *Public Health Nursing Services in Ireland Discussion Document*, Dublin.

Department of Justice, Equality and Law Reform (1996) *A Strategy for Equality, Report of the Commission on the Status of people with Disabilities*, Dublin.

Department of Justice, Equality and Law Reform (1999) *Towards Equal Citizenship: Progress Report on the Implementation of the Recommendations of the Commission on the Status of People with Disabilities*, Dublin.

Dick-Read, G. (1942) *Childbirth Without Fear*, Heinemann, London.

Dillon, P. (1997) *Breast or Bottle, Choice or Coercion?* unpublished MA in Women's Studies thesis, University College, Dublin.

Dinnerstein, D. (1987) *The Rocking of the Cradle and the Ruling of the World*, Women's Press, London.

Ditch, J., Bradshaw, J. and Eardley, T. (1997) *Developments in Family Policy in 1994*, European Observatory on National Family Policies, Social Policy Research Unit, York.

Dolan, M. (1996) *The Hepatitis C Handbook*, Catalyst Press, London.

Donnison, J. (1988) *Midwives and Medical Men: A History of the Struggle for the Control of Childbirth*, Historical Publications, Ltd., Herts and London (1st edition 1977 published by Heinemann).

Drake, R. (2001) *The Principles of Social Policy*, Basingstoke: Palgrave.

Drug Misuse Research Division (2002), *Trends in Treated Drug Misuse in the Eastern Health Board Area, 1996-1999*, Occasional Paper No.8/2002, HRB, Dublin.

Drugnet Newsletter of the Drug Misuse Research Division, Issue 4, Feb. 2002.

Dunlop, G. (1998) "The Home Birth Association of Ireland" in Kennedy, P. and Murphy Lawless, J. (eds.), *Returning Birth to Women: Challenging Policy and Practice*, Women's Education and Research Resource Centre, UCD and Centre for Women's Studies, TCD.

Eastern Health Board (1996) *Report of the Eastern Health Board Consultative Process on Women's Health*, Dublin.

Edwards, J. (1995) "Parenting Skills: Views of Community Health and Social Service Providers about the Needs of their 'Clients'", *Journal of Social Policy*, Vol. 24, pp. 237–314.

Ehrenreich, B. and English, D. (1973) *Witches, Midwives and Nurses: A History of Women's Bodies*, Feminist Press, New York.

EMCDDA (2000) *Annual Report on the State of the Drugs Problem in the European Union*, Office for Official Publications of the EU, Luxembourg.

EMCDDA (2001) *Annual Report on the State of the Drugs Problem in the European Union*, Office for Official Publications of the EU, Luxembourg.

Enkin, M., Marc, J.N.C., Keirse, J.N., Crowther, C., Duley, L., Hodnett, E. and Hofmeyr, J. (1995) *A Guide to Effective Care in Pregnancy and Childbirth*, Third edition, Oxford University Press, Oxford.

Esping-Anderson, G. (1990) *The Three Worlds of Welfare Capitalism*, Polity Press, Cambridge.

Evans, M. (1995) "Introduction" in Carter, P., *Feminism, Breasts and Breast-feeding*, Macmillan, London.

Fanning, B., Veale, A. and O'Connor, D. (2001) *Beyond the Pale: Asylum Seeking Children and Social Exclusion in Ireland*, Irish Refugee Council and the Combat Poverty Agency, Dublin.

Fanning, R. (1983) *Independent Ireland*, Helicon, Dublin.

Fanning, B. (1999) "The Mixed Economy of Welfare" in Quin, S., Kennedy, P., O'Donnell, A. and Kiely, G. (eds.), *Contemporary Irish Social Policy*, UCD Press, Dublin.

Fanning, B. (2002) "Revealing Poverty Amongst Asylum Seeking Children" *Poverty Today*, January, No. 53, Combat Poverty Agency, Dublin, pp. 4–5.

Farley, D. (1964) *Social Insurance and Social Assistance in Ireland*, Institute of Public Administration, Ireland.

Farmar, T. (1994) *Holles Street, 1894–1994, the National Maternity Hospital, A Centenary History*, A. & A. Farmar, Dublin.

Farrell, E. (2001) "Women, Children and Drug Use" in Moran, R, Dillon, L, O'Brien, M, Farrell, E and Pike, B (2001) *A Collection of Papers on Drug Issues in Ireland*, pp. 153–177, The Health Research Board, Dublin.

Faughnan, P., and O'Donovan, Á., (2002) *A Changing Voluntary Sector: Working with New Minority Communities in 2001: Summary of Findings*, Social Science Research Centre, UCD, Dublin.

Fawcett, B. (2000) *Feminist Perspectives on Disability*, Prentice Hall, Essex.

Feeney, J.K. (1950) *Clinical Report: Coombe Lying-In Hospital*, Dublin.

Fildes, V.A. (1988) *Wet Nursing: A History from Antiquity to the Present*, Basil Blackwell, Oxford.

Finch, J. and Groves, D. (eds.) (1983) *A Labour of Love: Women, Work and Caring*, Routledge and Kegan Paul, London.

Fine, M., and Asch, A., (1988) (eds.) *Women with Disabilities: Essays in Psychology, Culture and Politics*, Philadelphia, Temple University Press.

Finnegan, F. (2001) *Do Penance or Perish: A Study of Magdalen Asylums in Ireland*, Congrave Press, Piltown, Co. Kilkenny.

Firestone, S. (1979) *The Dialectic of Sex: The Case for Feminist Revolution*, Women's Press, London.

Fitzpatrick, C.C., Fitzpatrick, P.E. and Darling, M.R.N (1994) "Factors Associated with the Decision to Breastfeed among Irish Women", *Irish Medical Journal*, 87 (5), September/October.

Fitzpatrick, P., Molloy, B. and Johnson, Z. (1997) "Community Mothers' Programme: Extension to the Travelling Community in Ireland", *Journal of Epidemiology and Community Health*, 51, pp. 299–303.

Flanagan, N. and Richardson, V. (1992) *Unmarried Mothers: A Sociological Profile*, Department of Social Policy and Social Work/Social Work Research Unit, National Maternity Hospital, Dublin.

Flint, C. (1986) *Sensitive Midwifery*, Heinemann Medical Books, London.

Flint, C. and Poulengeris, P. (1987) *The Know Your Midwife Report*, 49 Peckarmans Wood, London, SE26 6RZ.

Ford, N. (2001) "A Review of Home Birth Services in Ireland", unpublished.

Foster, P. (1989) "Improving the Doctor/Patient Relationship: A Feminist Perspective", *Journal of Social Policy*, 18 (3), pp. 337–361.

Foster, P. (1995) *Women and the Health Care Industry: An Unhappy Relationship*, Open University Press, Buckingham.

Fraser, D. (1984) *The Evolution of the British Welfare State: A History of Social Policy*, Macmillan, Basingstoke.

French, S. (1993) "Disability, Impairment or Something in Between" in Swain, J., Finkelstein, V., French, S. and Oliver, M. (eds.), *Disabling Barriers — Enabling Environments*, OUP/Sage, London, pp. 17–25.

French, S. (1994a) "What is Disability?" in French, S. (ed.), *On Equal Terms: Working with Disabled People*, Butterworth Heinemann, Oxford pp. 3–16.

French, S. (1994b) "Dimensions of Disability and Impairment" in French, S. (ed.), *On Equal Terms: Working with Disabled People*, Butterworth Heinemann, Oxford, pp. 17–34.

Garcia, J. (1990) *The Politics of Maternity Care*, Clarendon Press, Oxford.

Gaskin, I.M. (1977) *Spiritual Midwifery*, The Book Publishing Company, Summertown, USA.

Glazener, C.M.A et al. (1995) "Postnatal Maternal Morbidity: Extent, Causes, Prevention and Treatment", *British Journal of Obstetrics and Gynaecology*, April, Vol. 102, pp. 282–287.

Glendinning, C. and Millar, J. (1992) *Women and Poverty in Britain* (2nd edition), Harvester Wheatsheaf, Hemel Hempstead.

Gordon, T. (1990) *Feminist Mothers*, Macmillan, Hampshire and London.

Gorham, D. and Kellner-Andrews, F. (1990) "The La Leche League: A Feminist Perspective" in Arnup, K., Levesque, A. and Pierson, R.R. (eds.), *Delivering Motherhood: Maternal Ideologies and Practises in the 19th and 20th Centuries*, Routledge, London.

Graham, H. (1983) "Caring: A Labour of Love" in Finch, J. and Groves, D. (eds.), *A Labour of Love*, Routledge and Kegan Paul, London.

Graham, H. (1995) "Cigarette Smoking: A Light on Gender and Class Inequality in Britain", *Journal of Social Policy*, Vol. 24, pp. 509–528.

Graham, H. and Oakley, A. (1981) "Competing Ideologies of Reproduction: Medical and Maternal Perspectives on Pregnancy" in Roberts, H. (ed.), *Women, Health and Reproduction*, RKP, London.

Greer, G. (1985) *Sex and Destiny: The Politics of Human Fertility*, Picador, London.

Griffin, S. (1984) *Woman and Nature: The Roaring Inside Her*, Women's Press, London.

Guilbride, A. (1996) "Mad or Bad? Women Committing Infanticide in Ireland from 1925–1957" in Lentin, R. (ed.), *In from the Shadows: The UL Women's Studies Collection*, Vol. II, Women's Studies/Department of Government and Society, University of Limerick.

Hardyment, C. (1983) *Dream Babies: Child Care from Locke to Spock*, Cape, London.

Hartmann, H. (1979) "The Unhappy Marriage of Marxism and Feminism: Towards a More Progressive Union", *Capital and Class*, No. 8; (revised) in Sargent, L. (ed.) (1981) *Women and Revolution*, Pluto Press, London and South End Press, Boston.

Hartmann, H. (ed.) (1985) *Comparable Worth: New Directions for Research*, National Academy Press, Washington.

Hartmann, H. and Treiman, D. (eds.) (1981) *Women, Work and Wages: Equal Pay for Equal Jobs of Equal Value*, National Academy Press, Washington.

Haughey, N. (2002a) "State contesting right of non-EU parents of Irish children to stay" in *The Irish Times*, 9 January 2002.

Haughey, N. (2002b) "Unique attitude to Irish citizens" in *The Irish Times*, 21 February 2002.

Haughey, N. (2002c) "Legal cases will test immigrant parents' status" in *The Irish Times*, 19 March 2002.

Hernes, H. (1987a) "Women and the Welfare State: The Transition from Private to Public Dependence" in Sassoon, A.S. (ed.), *Women and the State*, Hutchinson, London.

Hernes, H.M. (1987b) *Welfare State and Women Power*, Norwegian University Press, Oslo.

Hill, R. (1995) "Why do so few Irish Women Breastfeed?" in Lentin, R. (ed.), *In from the Shadows: The UL Women's Studies Collection*, Women's Studies/ Department of Government and Society, University of Limerick.

Hinds, B. (1991) "Child Care Provision and Policy" in Davies, C. and McLaughlin, E. (eds.), *Women, Employment and Social Policy in Northern Ireland: Problem Postponed?* Policy Research Institute, QUB and UU.

Holmes, J. (1993) *John Bowlby and Attachment Theory*, Routledge, London and New York.

Hopkins, S., Lyons, F., Mulcahy, F. and Bergin, C. (2001) "The Great Pretender Returns to Dublin, Ireland" in *SexTransf Infect* (Oct.), 77, 95, pp. 316-318.

House of Commons Health Committee (1992) *Maternity Services, Second Report, Vol. 1. Report together with Appendices and the Proceedings of the Committee*, HMSO, London.

Howe, D. (1995) *Attachment Theory and Social Work Practice*, Macmillan, London.

Howell, F., Bedford, B., O'Keeffe, B. and Corcoran, R. (1997) "Breastfeeding in a Health Board Region", *Irish Journal of Medical Science*, Vol. 166, Supplement No. 5.

Hunt, S. and Symonds, A. (1995) *The Social Meaning of Midwifery*, Macmillan: London.

Huntingford, P. (1978) "Obstetric Practice: Past, Present, and Future" in Kitzinger, S. and Davis, J. (eds.), *The Place of Birth*, Oxford University Press, Oxford:

Hutter, B. and Williams, G. (eds.) (1981) *Controlling Women*, Croom Helm, London.

Inch, S. (1981) *Birthrights: A Parent's Guide to Modern Childbirth*, Hutchinson, London.

Inch, S. (1990) "Post Natal Care Relating to Breastfeeding" in Alexander, J. Levy, V. and Roch, S. (eds.), *Post-natal Care: A Research-based Approach*, Macmillan, London.

Inciardi, J. and Harrison, C.D. (2000) *Harm Reduction: National and International Perspectives*, London, Sage.

Irish Council for Civil Liberties (ICCL) (2000) *Women and the Refugee Experience: Towards a Statement of Best Practice*, Dublin.

Irish National Coordinating Committee for the European Year Against Racism (1997), "The Framework Programme for the European Year Against Racism 1997", Dublin.

Jackson, P. (1987a) "Outside the Jurisdiction: Irish Women Seeking Abortion", in Curtin, C., Jackson, P. and O'Connor, B., *Gender in Irish Society*, Galway University Press, Galway, pp. 203–223.

Jackson, P. (1987b) *Migrant Women: The Republic of Ireland*, Department of Social Science, UCD.

Jackson, R. (1994) *Mothers Who Leave: Behind the Myth of Women without their Children*, Pandora, London.

Jelliffe, D.B. and Jelliffe, P. (1978) *Human Milk in the Modern World: Psychosocial, Nutritional and Economic Significance*, Oxford University Press, Oxford.

Johnson, N. (1987) *The Welfare State in Transition*, Harvester Wheatsheaf, London.

Johnson, Z. and Molloy, B. (1995) "The Community Mothers Programme: Empowerment of Parents by Parents", *Children and Society*, 9 (2), pp. 73–85.

Johnson, Z., Molloy, B. and Howell, F. (1993) "Community Mothers Programme: Randomised Controlled Trial of Non-Professional Intervention in Parenting", *British Medical Journal*, May, Vol. 306, pp. 1149–1452.

Johnston, M. (1985) *Around the Banks of Pimlico*, Attic, Dublin.

Kaim-Caudle, P. (1967) *Social Policy in the Irish Republic*, Routledge and Kegan Paul, London.

Kane, H. (2000) "Leaving Home: The Flow of Refugees" in Cusimano, M. (ed.), *Beyond Sovereignty: Issues for a Global Agenda*, Bedford/St. Martin's Press, New York.

Kaplan, M. (1991) *Images of the Mother*, Routledge, New York.

Keenan, E., Dorman, A., and O'Connor, J.J. (1993) "Six Year Follow-up Study of Forty-five Pregnant Opiate Addicts", *Irish Journal of Medical Science*, 162: pp. 252–255.

Keirse, M. (1989a) "Social and Professional Support During Childbirth" in Chalmers, I. et al. (eds.), *Effective Care in Pregnancy and Childbirth*, Oxford University Press, Oxford.

Keirse, M. (1989b) "Augmentation of Labour" in Chalmers, I. et al. (eds.), *Effective Care in Pregnancy and Childbirth*, Oxford University Press, Oxford.

Kennedy, F. (1994) *Challenges for Family Policies for the Future*, Paper for Seminar *Family Income Support in Ireland — 50 Years On*, Department of Social Welfare and European Institute of Social Security (Irish Branch), Dublin Castle, 23 September..

Kennedy, P. (1984) *The Development of Youth Work Services and Policy in Ireland*, unpublished M.Soc.Sc. Thesis, University College Cork.

Kennedy, P. (1997) "A Comparative Study of Maternity Entitlements in Ireland and Northern Ireland" in Byrne, A. and Leonard, M. (eds.), *Women and Irish Society: A Sociological Reader*, Beyond the Pale, Belfast, pp. 311–324.

Kennedy, P. (1998) "Between the Lines", in Kennedy, P. and Murphy-Lawless, J. (eds.), *Returning Birth to Women: Challenging Policy and Practice*, Women's Education and Research Resource Centre, UCD, and Centre for Women's Studies, TCD.

Kennedy. P. (1999) "Women and Social Policy" in Kiely, G., O'Donnell, G., Kennedy, P. and Quin, S. (eds.), *Irish Social Policy in Context*, UCD Press, Dublin, pp. 231–253.

Kennedy, P. (2001) "Travellers in Ireland: Training and Health Issues — Lessons for Social Policy" in *RDD Regional Development Dialogue*, UN Centre for Regional Development, Spring 2001, Vol. 22, No. 1, pp. 79–90.

Kennedy, P. and Murphy-Lawless, J. (eds.) (1998) *Returning Birth to Women: Challenging Policy and Practice*, Women's Education and Research Resource Centre, UCD, and Centre for Women's Studies, TCD.

Kennedy, P. and Murphy-Lawless, J. (2002) *The Maternity Care Needs of Refugee and Asylum-seeking Women: A Research Study Conducted for the Women's Health Unit*, Dublin, Northern Area Health Authority.

Keogh, F.A. (2002) "Pregnancy, Heroin Addiction and Social Work", M.Soc.Sc. Social work thesis, UCD.

Kiely, G. (1995) "Fathers in Families" in McCarthy, I.C. (ed.), *Irish Family Studies: Selected Papers*, Family Studies Centre, UCD.

Kiely, G (2002) "General Monitoring Report 1996–2001: Ireland" in *EU Observatory of Demography, the Social Situation and the Family*, Austrian Institute of Family Studies, Oslo.

Kirkham, M. (1989) "Midwives and Information-Giving During Labour" in Robinson, S. and Thompson, A.M. (eds.), *Midwives, Research and Childbirth*, Chapman Hall, London.

Kitzinger, S. (1972) *The Experience of Childbirth* (3rd edition), Penguin, Harmondsworth.

Kitzinger, S. (1977) *Education and Counselling for Childbirth*, Ballière Tindall, London.

Kitzinger, S. (1978) *Women as Mothers*, Fontana, Great Britain.

Kitzinger, S. (1979) *The Experience of Breastfeeding*, Penguin, Middlesex.

Kitzinger, S. (1984) *The Experience of Childbirth*, Penguin, London.

Kitzinger, S. (1983) *Women's Experience of Sex*, Penguin, London.

Kitzinger, S. (1988) "Why Women Need Midwives", in Kitzinger, S. (ed), *The Midwife Challenge*, Pandora Press, London.

Kitzinger, S. (1992) *Giving Birth: How it Really Feels*, Victor Gollancz, London.

Kitzinger, S. (1993) *Ourselves as Mothers*, Bantam, London.

Kitzinger, S. (1994) *The Year After Childbirth*, Oxford University Press, Oxford. .

Kitzinger, S. (1995) *Home Births and Other Alternatives to Hospital*, Dorling Kindersley, London.

Kitzinger, J. (1997) "Sexual Violence and Midwifery Practice" in Karger, I. and Hunt, S.C., *Challenges in Midwifery Care*, Macmillan, Basingstoke.

Kitzinger, S. and Davis, J. (eds.) (1978) *The Place of Birth*, Oxford University Press, Oxford.

Klaus, M.H., Trauses, M.A. and Kennell, J.H. (1975) "Does Human Maternal Behaviour after Delivery show a Characteristic Pattern?", *Parent–Infant Interaction*, Ciba Foundation Symposium 33 (New Series) (69–78), Elsevier, Amsterdam.

Klaus, M.H. and Kennell, J.H. (1982) *Maternal Infant Bonding* (2nd ed.) Mosby, Saint Louis.

Klein, M. (1981) *Love, Guilt and Reparation*, Hogarth Press, London.

Klein, R. (1993) "O'Goffe's Tale, or what we can learn from the success of the capitalist welfare states?" in Jones, C. (ed.) *New Perspectives on the Welfare State in Europe*, Routledge, London.

La Leche League International (1981) *The Womanly Art of Breastfeeding*, La Leche League International, USA.

La Leche League of Ireland (1992) *Breastfeeding: The Best Beginning*, Dublin.

Lamaze, F. (1958) *Painless Childbirth: Psychoprophylatic Techniques*, Burke, London.

Leboyer, F. (1991) *Birth Without Violence* (2nd ed.; 1st edition 1975), Mandarin, London.

Leboyer, F. (1997) *Loving Hands*, Collins, London.

Lee, J.J. (1989) *Ireland, 1912–1985: Politics and Society*, Cork University Press, Cork.

Leira, A. (1992) *Welfare States and Working Mothers*, Cambridge University Press, Cambridge.

Leira, A. (1993) "Mothers, Markets and the State: A Scandinavian Model?" *Journal of Social Policy*, 22 (3), pp. 329–347.

Leira, A. (1994) "Concepts of Caring, Loving, Thinking and Doing", *Social Service Review*, June, pp. 85–201.

Leonard, M. (1997) "Caring and Sharing in Belfast", in Byrne, A. and Leonard, M. (eds.) *Women and Irish Society: A Sociological Reader*, Beyond the Pale, Belfast, pp. 111–126.

Lerner, G. (1986) *The Creation of Patriarchy*, Open University Press, London.

Levy, V., Robinson, S. and Thomson, A.M. (eds.) (1993) *Midwives, Research and Childbirth*, Vol. 3, Chapman and Hall, London.

Lewis, J. (1992) "Gender and the Development of Welfare Regimes", *Journal of European Social Policy*, 2 (3), pp. 159–173.

Lewis, J. (ed.) (1993) *Women and Social Policies in Europe: Work, Family and the State*, Edward Elgar, New York.

Lewis, J. (ed.) (1997) *Lone Mothers in European Welfare Regimes: Shifting Policy Logics*, Jessica Kingsley, London.

Littlewood, J. and McHugh, N. (1997) *Maternal Distress and Postnatal Depression: The Myth of Madonna*, Macmillan, London.

Lois, K. and Morris, J. (1996) "Easy Targets: A Disability Rights Perspective on the Children as Carers Debate" in Morris, J. (1996) (ed.), *Encounters with Strangers: Feminism and Disability — The Major Issue Confronting Feminism Today*, The Women's Press, London, pp. 89–115.

Lowry, M. and Lillis, D.F. (1993) "Infant Feeding Practises", *The Irish Medical Journal*, Vol. 86, No 7, pp. 13–14.

Lynch, K. and McLaughlin, E. (1995) "Caring Labour and Love Labour", in Clancy, P., Drudy, S. Lynch, K. and O'Dowd, L. (eds.), *Irish Society: Sociological Perspectives*, Institute of Public Administration, Dublin, pp. 250–292.

Lyons, F.S.L. (1973) *Ireland Since the Famine*, Collins, Suffolk.

MacAdam-O'Connell, B. (1998) "Risk, Responsibility and Choice: The Medical Model of Birth and Alternatives" in Kennedy, P. and Murphy-Lawless, J. (eds.), *Returning Birth to Women: Challenging Policy and Practice*, Women's Education and Research Resource Centre, UCD, and Centre for Women's Studies, TCD.

McCarthy, A. (1997) *The Enniscorthy Lunatic Asylum*, unpublished MA (Women's Studies) Thesis, WERRC, UCD.

McCarthy, A. (2000) "Sexual Violence against Refugee Women" in UNHCR (ed.), *Refugee Women — Victims or Survivors?* UNHCR, Dublin.

McCarthy, I.C. (1995a) "Introduction" in McCarthy, I.C. (ed.), *Irish Family Studies: Selected Papers*, Family Studies Centre, University College, Dublin.

McCarthy, I.C. (1995b) "Women Poverty and Systemic Family Therapy", in McCarthy, I.C. (ed.), *Irish Family Studies: Selected Papers*, Family Studies Centre, University College, Dublin.

McCarton, C.M., Wallace, I.F. and Bennett, F.C. (1995) "Preventative Interventions with Low Birth Weight Premature Infants: An Evaluation of Their Success", *Seminars in Perinatalogy*, Vol. 19, No. 4 (August), pp. 330–340.

McCluskey, D., O'Keeffe, M. and Slattery, S. (1996) *The Child Health Care Service, Mothers' Views,* The Institute of Community Health Nursing

MacCurtain, M. (1978) "Women, the Vote and Revolution", in MacCurtain, M. and O'Corrain, D., *Women in Irish Society: The Historical Dimension,* Arlen House, Dublin, pp. 46–57.

MacCurtain, M. and O'Corrain, D. (1978) *Women in Irish Society: The Historical Dimension,* Arlen House, Dublin.

MacCurtain, M. and O'Dowd, M. (1991) *Women in Early Modern Ireland,* Edinburgh University Press, Edinburgh.

McLaughlin, E. (1993) "Ireland: Catholic Corporatism" in Cochrane, A. and Clarke, J. (eds.), *Comparing Welfare States: Britain in an International Context,* Open University, Sage, London.

McLeish, J. (2002) *Mothers in Exile: Maternity Experiences of Asylum Seekers in England,* Maternity Alliance, London.

McSweeney, M. and Kevany, J. (1982) *Infant Feeding Practices in Ireland,* Health Education Bureau, Dublin. (This study was carried out in the Human Nutrition Unit, Department of Community Health in Trinity College Dublin, completed in July, 1982).

McSweeney, M. and Kevany, J. (1983) *National Survey of Infant Feeding Practices,* Health Education Bureau, Dublin.

McSweeney, M. and Kevany, J. (1986) *National Survey of Infant Feeding Practices,* Health Education Bureau, Dublin.

Maguire, M. (1986) "Ireland" in Flora, P. (ed.), *Growth to Limits: The Western European Welfare States since World War II,* Vol. 2, Walter de Gruyter, Berlin.

Maher, V. (1992) "Breast-feeding in Cross-cultural Perspective" in Maher, V. (ed.), *The Anthropology of Breast-feeding: Natural Law or Social Construct,* Berg, Oxford.

Mahon, E. (1987) "Women's Rights and Catholicism in Ireland", *New Left Review,* No. 166, Nov/Dec, pp. 53–77.

Mahon, E., Conlon, C. and Dillon, L. (1998) *Women and Crisis Pregnancy,* Stationery Office, Dublin.

Manning, M. (1987) *The Blueshirts,* Gill and Macmillan, Dublin.

Martin, D. (1998) "Cuidiú: The Irish Childbirth Trust" in Kennedy, P. and Murphy-Lawless, J. (eds.) *Returning Birth to Women: Challenging Policy and Practice*, Women's Education and Research Resource Centre, UCD, and Centre for Women's Studies, TCD.

Mason, M. (1995) *Towards Woman-Centred Childbirth through Childbirth Education*, Unpublished MA (Women's Studies) Thesis, University College, Dublin.

Mason, M. (1998) "Hospital-Based Childbirth Education: In Whose Interests?" in Kennedy, P. and Murphy-Lawless, J. (eds.) *Returning Birth to Women: Challenging Policy and Practice*, Women's Education and Research Resource Centre, UCD, and Centre for Women's Studies, TCD.

Maternity Alliance (1993a) *Mothers Pride and Others Prejudice: A Survey of Disabled Mothers' Experience of Maternity*, Maternity Alliance, London.

Maternity Alliance (1993b) *Listen to us for a Change: A Charter for Disabled Parents and Parents to Be*, Maternity Alliance, London.

Mayall, B. (1990) "The Division of Labour in Early Child Care — Mothers and Others", *Journal of Social Policy*, 19 (3), pp. 229–330.

Meire, H. (1987) "The Safety of Diagnostic Ultrasound", *British Journal of Obstetrics and Gynaecology*, Vol. 94, pp. 1121–1122.

Methven, R. (1989) "Recording an Obstetric History or Relating to a Pregnant Woman? A Study of the Ante-natal booking interview" in Robinson, S. and Thomson, A.M. (eds.), *Midwives, Research and Childbirth*, Vol. 1, Chapman and Hall, London.

Methven, R.C. (1990) "The Antenatal Booking Interview" in Alexander, J., Levy, V. and Roch, S. (eds.), *Post-natal Care: A Research-Based Approach*, Macmillan, London.

Milner, M., Beckett, M., Coghlan, D., Matthews, T.G., McNally, M., Clarke, T.A., Lambert, I. and McDermott, C. (1999) "Neonatal Abstinence Syndrome", *IMJ*, Jan/Feb, Vol. 92, No. 1.

Mills, F. (1991) *The Scheme of Last Resort*, Combat Poverty Agency, Dublin.

Milotte, M. (1997) *Banished Babies: The Secret History of Ireland's Baby Export Business*, New Island Books, Dublin.

Ministry of Health (1970) *Domiciliary Midwifery and Maternity Bed Needs: The Report of the Standing Maternity and Advisory Committee*, Peel, J. (Chairman), HMSO, London.

Moran, J. (1999) "Refugees and Social Policy" in Quin, S. et al. (eds.), *Contemporary Irish Social Policy*, UCD Press, Dublin.

Moran, R., Dillon, L., O'Brien, M., Farrell, E. and Pike, B. (2001) *A Collection of Papers on Drug Issues in Ireland*, The Health Research Board, Dublin.

Moran, R., O'Brien, M., Dillon, L., Farrell, E. and Mayock, P. (2001) *Overview of Drug Issues in Ireland 2000*, Drug Misuse Research Division, HRB, Dublin

Morris, J. (ed.) (1989) *Able Lives Women's Experience of Paralysis*, Women's Press, London.

Morris, J. (1993) "Feminism and Disability", *Feminist Review*, No. 43, Spring.

Morris, J. (1993) *Pride against Prejudice* (2nd ed.), Women's Press, London.

Morris, J. (1994) "Gender and Disability" in French, S. (ed.) *On Equal Terms: Working with Disabled People*, pp. 207–219, Butterworth Heinemann, Oxford.

Morris, J. (1995) "Creating a Space for Feminist Voices: Disabled Women's Experiences of Receiving Assistance with Daily Living Activities", *Feminist Review*, No. 51, Autumn, pp. 68–93.

Morris, J. (ed.) (1996) *Encounters with Strangers: Feminism and Disability — The Major Issue Confronting Feminism Today*, Women's Press, London.

Morris, J. (1997) "'Us' and 'Them'? Feminist Research, Community Care and Disability" in Taylor, D. (ed.), *Critical Social Policy*, Sage, London, pp. 77–94.

Muecke, M. (1992) "New Paradigms for Refugee Health Problems", *Social Science and Medicine*, Vol. 35, No. 4, pp. 515–523.

Murphy, J.F.A. (2000) "The Drug Problem in the European Union", *IMJ Commentary 2000*, Vol. 93, No. 9.

Murphy-Black, T. (1990) "Antenatal Education" in Alexander, J., Levy, V. and Roch, S. (eds.), *Antenatal Care: A Research-Based Approach*, Macmillan, London.

Murphy-Lawless, J. (1987) *Women in Childbirth: The Invention of Female Incompetence*, unpublished PhD thesis, Dublin University, Trinity College, Dublin.

Murphy-Lawless, J. (1988) "The Obstetric View of Feminine Identity: A Case History of the Use of Forceps on Unmarried Women in 19th-Century Ireland", Todd and Fisher (eds.), *Gender and Discourse: The Power of Talk*, Ablex, Norwood, NJ.

Murphy-Lawless, J. (1991a) "Images of 'Poor Women' in the Writings of Irish Men Midwives", MacCurtain, M. and O'Dowd, M. (eds.), *Women in Early Modern Ireland*, Edinburgh University Press, Edinburgh.

Murphy-Lawless, J. (1991b) "Piggy in the Middle: The midwife's Role in Achieving Woman-Controlled Childbirth", *Irish Journal of Psychology*, Vol. 12, No. 2, pp. 198–215.

Murphy-Lawless, J. (1992a) "Reading Birth and Death through Obstetric Practice", *Canadian Journal of Irish Studies*, Vol. 18, No. 1, pp. 129–145.

Murphy-Lawless, J. (1992b) "The Obstetric View of Feminine Identity: A Nineteenth-Century Case History of the Use of Forceps in Ireland" in Smyth, A. (ed), *The Abortion Papers*, Attic Press, Dublin.

Murphy-Lawless, J. (1993a) "The Silencing of Women in Childbirth" in Smyth, A. (ed.), *Irish Women's Studies Reader*, Attic Press, Dublin.

Murphy-Lawless, J. (1993b) "Fertility, Bodies and Politics: The Irish Case", *Reproductive Health Matters*, No. 2, Nov., pp. 53–64.

Murphy-Lawless, J. (1998a) *Reading Birth and Death: A History of Obstetric Thinking*, Cork University Press, Cork.

Murphy-Lawless, J. (1998b) "Women Dying in Childbirth: Safe Motherhood in the International Context" in Kennedy, P. and Murphy-Lawless, J. (eds.) *Returning Birth to Women: Challenging Policy and Practice*, Women's Education and Research Resource Centre, UCD and Centre for Women's Studies, TCD.

Murphy-Lawless, J. (2002) *Fighting Back: Women and the Impact of Drug Abuse on Families and Communities*, The Liffey Press, Dublin.

Murray, B. and O'Carroll, A. (1997) "Out of Sight, Out of Mind? Women with Disabilities in Ireland" in Byrne, A. and Leonard, M. (eds.) *Women and Irish Society: A Sociological Reader*, Beyond the Pale, Belfast, pp. 494–512.

Nankano, G.E. (1994) "Social Constructions of Mothering: A Thematic Overview", in Nankano, G.E., Chang, G. and Rennie Forcey, L., *Mothering, Ideology, Experience and Agency*, Routledge, London.

National Childbirth Trust, *Resource List: A Parent Ability Guide to Pregnancy, Birth and Parenthood for People with Disabilities*, NCT, London.

National Childcare Strategy Report of the Partnership 2000 Expert Working Group on Childcare, Jan., Stationery Office, Dublin.

National Children's Strategy (2000) *Our Children — Their Lives*, Stationery Office, Dublin.

National Economic and Social Forum (1996) *Equality Proofing Issues*, Forum Report, No. 10, NESF, Dublin.

National Economic and Social Forum (2002) *A Strategic Policy Framework for Equality Issues*, Forum Report, No. 23, NESF, Dublin.

National Maternity Hospital, *Annual Clinical Reports* 1970–2000 (30 Reports).

National Public Health Nursing Committee (1994) *A Service Without Walls: An Analysis of Public Health Nursing in Ireland*, Dublin.

Neeson, D. (1995) (ed.) *A Consumer's Guide to Maternity Units in Ireland* (2nd ed.), Irish Association for Improvements in Maternity Services, Health Promotion Unit, Department of Health, Dublin.

Newberger, E.H., Barken, S.E. and Lieberman, E.S. (1992) "Abuse of Pregnant Women and Adverse Birth Outcome: Current Knowledge and Implications for Practice", *Journal of the American Medical Association*, 267, pp. 121–123.

Nic Ghiolla Phadraig (1994) "Daycare: Adult Interest Versus Children's Need? A Question of Compatability" in Qvortrup, J. (eds.), *Childhood Matters*, Avebury, Aldershot.

Nugent, J.K. et al. (1991) "Neurobehavioural and Medical Effects of Prenatal Alcohol and Cigarette Use", *Irish Journal of Psychology*, 12 (2), pp. 153–210.

Nutrition Advisory Group (1995) *Recommendations for a Food and Nutrition Policy for Ireland*, Government of Ireland, Dublin.

Oakley, A. (1974) *The Sociology of Housework*, Martin Robertson, London.

Oakley, A. (1976) "Wisewoman and Medicine Man" in Mitchell, J. and Oakley, A. (eds.), *The Rights and Wrongs of Women*, Penguin, Harmondsworth.

Oakley, A. (1979) *Becoming a Mother*, Martin Robertson, London.

Oakley, A. (1980) *Women Confined: Towards a Sociology of Childbirth*, Martin Robertson, Oxford.

Oakley, A. (1981a) "Interviewing Women: A Contradiction in Terms?" in Roberts, H. (ed.), *Doing Feminist Research*, Routledge and Kegan Paul, London.

Oakley, A. (1981b) "Normal Motherhood: An Exercise in Social Control? in Hutter, B. and Williams, G. (eds.), *Controlling Women*, Croom Helm, London.

Oakley, A. (1986a) "Feminism, Motherhood and Medicine: Who Cares?" in Oakley, A. and Mitchell, J. (eds.), *What is Feminism?*, Blackwell, Oxford.

Oakley, A. (1986b) *The Captured Womb: A History of the Medical Care of Pregnant Women* (2nd edition), Basil Blackwell, Oxford.

Oakley, A. (1992) *Social Support and Motherhood: The Natural History*, Blackwell, Oxford.

Oakley, A. (1993) *Essays on Women, Medicine and Health*, Edinburgh University Press, Edinburgh.

Oakley, A., McPherson, A. and Roberts, H. (1984) *Miscarriage*, Fontana, Glasgow.

O'Brien, M. (1981) *The Politics of Reproduction*, RKP, London.

O'Brien, M. and Dillon, L. (2001) "Health Issues and Consequences of Drug Misuse", in Moran, R., O'Brien, M., Dillon, L., Farrell, E. and Mayock, P., *Overview of Drug Issues in Ireland 2000*, Drug Misuse Research Division, HRB, Dublin, pp. 55–78.

O'Brien, M., Kelleher, T. and Cahill, P. (2002) *Trends in Treated Drug Misuse in the Eastern Health Board Area 1996–1999*, Occasional Paper No. 8/2002, Drug Misuse Research Division.

O'Campo, P., Davis, M.V. and Gielen, A.C. (1995) "Smoking Cessation Interventions for Pregnant Women: Review and Future Directions", *Seminars in Perinatalogy*, Vol. 19, No. 4 (August), pp. 279–285.

O'Connor, M. (1992) *Women and Birth: A National Study of Intentional Home Births in Ireland*, study conducted under the aegis of the Coombe Lying-In Hospital and the Department of Health, Dublin.

O'Connor, M. (1995) *Birth Tides*, Pandora, London.

O'Connor, M. (1998) "Redefining Risk: Life, Death and Home Birth", in Kennedy, P. and Murphy-Lawless, J. (eds.), *Returning Birth to Women: Challenging Policy and Practice*, Women's Education and Research Resource Centre, UCD, and Centre for Women's Studies, TCD.

O'Connor, P. (1999) *Parents Supporting Parents: An Evaluation Report on the National Parent Support Programme Mid-West*, National Parent Support Mid-West, Mid Western Health Board and University of Limerick.

Odent, M. (1991) *Birth Reborn* (2nd ed.; 1st ed. 1984), Pantheon, New York.

O'Dowd, L. (1986) "Beyond Industrial Society" in Clancy, P., Drudy, S., Lynch, K. and O'Dowd, L. (eds.), *Ireland: A Sociological Profile*, Institute of Public Administration, Dublin, pp. 198–221.

O'Driscoll, K., Meagher, D. and Boylan, P. (1993) *Active Management of Labour: The Dublin Experience* (3rd ed.; 2nd ed. 1986), The National Maternity Hospital and UCD, Mosby Year Book Europe, Limited.

Ó Gráda, C. (1997) *A Rocky Road: The Irish Economy Since the 1920s*, Manchester University Press, Manchester.

O'Hagan, J.W. (1975) *The Economy of Ireland: Policy and Performance*, Irish Management Institute, Dublin.

O'Kelly, A. (1998) "Still Outside the Circle: The Experience of Irish Women with Disabilities" in Barry, M., Conroy, J., Hayes, A., O'Kelly, A. and Shaughnessy, L. (eds.), *Women's Studies Review*, Volume V, Women's Studies Centre, National University of Ireland, Galway, pp. 91–110.

Oliver, M. (1996) *Understanding Disability: From Theory to Practice*, London: Macmillan.

O'Meara, C. (1993) "Childbirth and Parenting Education: The Providers' Viewpoint", *Midwifery*, 9, pp. 76–84.

O'Regan, M. (1998) "Totalitarian Maternity Care: Obstacles to Fully Establishing Women's Autonomy in Maternity Care" in Kennedy, P. and Murphy-Lawless, J. (eds.), *Returning Birth to Women: Challenging Policy and Practice*, Women's Education and Research Resource Centre, UCD, and Centre for Women's Studies, TCD.

Pahl, J. (1990) "Household Spending, Personal Spending and the Control of Money in Marriage", *Sociology*, Vol. 24, No. 1, pp. 119–138.

Palmer, G. (1988) *The Politics of Breastfeeding*, Pandora, London.

Parish, S.L. (2002) "Parenting" in Walsh Noonan, P. and Heller, T. (2002), *Health of Women with Intellectual Disabilities*, Blackwell, Oxford.

Patchen, L. and Beal, M.W. (2001) "Preventing Perinatal Transmission of HIV: An Evidence-Based Update for Midwives", *Journal of Midwifery and Women's Health*, Vol. 46, No. 6, November/December, American College of Nurse-Midwives, Elsevier Science Inc., pp. 354–365.

Pateman, C. (1988) "The Patriarchal Welfare State" in Gutman, A. (ed.), *Democracy and the Welfare State*, Princeton University Press, Princeton.

Pavee Point and Eastern Health Board (2000) *Primary Health Care for Travellers Project, Implementation Report 1996–1999*, Pavee Point Publications, Dublin.

Pavee Point Travellers' Centre (2002) *Traveller Proofing — Within an Equality Framework*, Pavee Point Travellers Centre, Dublin.

Petchesky, R. (1986) *Abortion and Woman's Choice: The State, Sexuality and Reproductive Freedom*, Verso, London.

Peterson, G.H. and Mehl, L.E. (1978) "Some Determinants of Maternal Attachment", *American Journal of Psychiatry*, Vol. 135, pp. 1168–1173.

Pigot, M. (1996) *Coping with Post-natal Depression: Light at the End of the Tunnel*, Columba Press, Dublin.

Pitts, T. (1998) *Women and Epilepsy*, Martin Dunitz, UK.

Pius XI (1930) *Casti Connubi*, Papal Encylical, 31 December.

Pius XI (1931) *Quadragesimo Anno*, Papal Encyclical, 15 May.

Porter, M. and MacIntyre, S. (1989) "Psychosocial Effectiveness of Ante-natal and Post-natal Care" in Robinson, S. and Thomson, A.M. (eds.), *Midwives, Research and Childbirth*, Vol. 1, Chapman and Hall, London.

Powell, F.W. (1992) *The Politics of Irish Social Policy, 1600–1900*, Edwin Mellen Press, New York.

Price, A. and Price, B. (1993) "Midwifery Knowledge: Theory for Action, Theory for Practice", *The British Journal of Midwifery*, Vol. 1, No. 5, pp. 233–237.

Primary Health Care for Travellers Project (1996) *Project Report for Year Ended October 1995*, Pavee Point and Eastern Health Board, Pavee Point Publications, Dublin.

Proud, J. (1989) "Placental Grading: A Test of Fetal Well-Being", in Robinson, S. and Thomson, A.M. (eds.), *Midwives, Research and Childbirth*, Vol. 1, Chapman and Hall, London.

Proud, J. (1990) "The Midwife's Role," in Alexander, J., Levy, V. and Roch, S. (eds.), *Ante-natal Care: A Research-Based Approach*, Macmillan, Basingstoke.

Proud, J. (1994) *Understanding Obstetric Ultrasound: A Guide for Midwives and Health Professionals*, Books for Midwives Press, Cheshire, England.

Quin, S. and Redmond, B. (1999) "Moving from Needs to Rights: Social Policy for People with Disability in Ireland" in Quin, S. et al. (eds.), *Contemporary Irish Social Policy*, UCD Press, Dublin, pp. 146–165.

Quinlan, F. (2002) "State to Fight Rights of Refugee Parents", *The Examiner*, 22 February.

Quirke, B., "Traveller Proofing Health" in *Traveller Proofing within an Equality Framework*, Pavee Point Travellers Centre, Dublin, pp. 6–11.

Randall, V. (1996) "Feminism and Daycare", *Journal of Social Policy*, Vol. 25, pp. 485–507.

Raphael, D. (1973) *The Tender Gift, Breastfeeding*, Prentice Hall, London.

Redmond, B. (1996) *Listening to Parents: The Aspirations, Expectations, and Anxieties of Parents about Their Teenagers with Learning Disability*, Family Studies Centre, UCD, Dublin.

Refugee Women's Legal Group (1998) "Gender Guidelines for the Adjudication of Female Asylum Claimants in the UK".

Reinharz, S. (1992) *Feminist Methods in Social Research*, Open University Press, Milton Keynes.

Report of the Commission on the Status of People with Disabilities: A Strategy for Equality (1996), Stationery Office, Dublin.

Report of the Working Group on Childcare Facilities for Working Parents (1994), Stationery Office, Dublin.

Report of the Working Party on the General Medical Service (1994), Stationery Office, Dublin.

Reproductive Health for Refugees Consortium (1998) *Refugees and Reproductive Health: The Next Step*, New York.

Rich, A. (1977) *Of Woman Born: Motherhood as Experience and Institution*, Virago, London.

Rich, A. (1980) *On Lies, Secrets and Silence: Selected Prose 1966-1978*, Virago, London.

Richardson, D. (1993) *Women, Motherhood and Childrearing*, Macmillan, London.

Roberts, H. (ed.) (1981) *Doing Feminist Research*, Routledge and Kegan Paul, London.

Robertson, A. (1994) *Empowering Women: Teaching Active Birth in the '90s*, ACE Graphics, Australia.

Robins, J. (2000) *Nursing and Midwifery in Ireland in the Twentieth Century*, An Bord Altranais, Dublin.

Robinson, M. (1978) "Women and the New Irish State" in MacCurtain, M. and O'Corrain, D., *Women in Irish Society: The Historical Dimension*, Arlen House, Dublin.

Robinson, V. and Richardson, D. (eds.) (1997) *Introducing Women's Studies*, Macmillan, London.

Robson, M. and Kumar, R. (1980) "Delayed Onset of Maternal Affection after Childbirth", *British Journal of Psychiatry*, Vol. 136, pp. 347–353.

Rogers, J. and Matsumura, M. (1991) *Mother To Be: A Guide to Pregnancy and Birth for Women with Disabilities*, Demos Publications, New York.

Rottman, D. (1994) *Income Distribution in Irish Households,* Combat Poverty Agency, Dublin.

Rotunda Hospital, *Annual Clinical Reports,* 1970–2000, Dublin (30 Reports).

Royston, E. and Armstrong, S. (1989) *Preventing Maternal Deaths,* WHO, Geneva.

Ruggie, M. (1984) *The State and Working Women,* Princeton University Press, Princeton.

Rutter, M. (1972) *Maternal Deprivation Reassessed,* Penguin, London.

Ryan, S. (1997) "Interventions in Childbirth: The Midwives Role", in Byrne, A. and Leonard, M. (eds.) *Women and Irish Society: A Sociological Reader,* Beyond the Pale, Belfast, pp. 255–267.

Ryan, S.C., Griffin, E., Kelly, M.G., Magee, T. and Stafford-Johnson, S. (1983) "The Emergence of Maternal Drug Addiction as a Problem in Ireland", *Irish Medical Journal,* Feb., Vol. 76, No. 2.

Sachs, L. (2000) "Sexual Violence as a Tool of War" in UNHCR (ed.) *Refugee Women: Victims or Survivors?* UNHCR, Dublin.

Sainsbury, D. (ed.) (1994) *Gendering Welfare States,* Sage, London.

Santmyire, B.R. (2001) "Vertical Transmission of HIV from Mother to Child in Sub-Saharan Africa: Modes of Transition and Methods for Prevention". *Obstetrical and Gynaecological Survey,* Vol. 56, No. 5. pp. 306–312.

Saorstát Éireann (1927) *Report of the Commission on the Relief of the Sick and Destitute Poor, Including the Insane Poor,* Stationery Office, Dublin.

Sayers, G., Thornton, L., Corcoran, R. and Burke, M. (1995) "Influences on Breastfeeding Initiation and Duration", *Irish Journal of Medical Science,* Vol. 164, No. 4, Oct–Dec.

Sayers, J. (1982) *Biological Politics, Feminist and Anti-feminist Perspectives,* Tavistock, London.

Sayers, J., Deutsch, D., Horney, K., Freud, A. and Klein, M. (eds.) (1991) *Mothering Psychoanalysis,* Hamish, London.

Sayers, J., Evans, M. and Redclift, N. (eds.) (1987) *Engels Revisited: New Feminist Essays,* Tavistock, London.

Scanlan, P. (1991) *The Irish Nurse — A Study of Nursing in Ireland: History and Education 1718–1981,* Drumlin Publications, County Leitrim.

Scarrow, S.E. (2001) "Obstetrical Delivery of the HIV-Positive Woman: Legal and Ethical Considerations", *Obstetrical and Gynecological Survey*, Vol. 56, No. 3, Lippincott Williams and Wilkins, Inc., pp. 178–183.

Schaefer, C., Coyne, J.C. and Lazarus, R.S. (1981) "The Health-related Functions of Social Support", *Journal of Behavioural Medicine*, 4 (4), pp. 381–405.

Scheiwe, K. (1994) "Labour Market, Welfare State and Family Institutions: The Links to Mothers' Poverty Risks: A Comparison between Belgium, Germany and the United Kingdom", *Journal of European Social Policy*, 4 (3), pp. 201–224.

Second Commission on the Status of Women: Report to Government (1993), Stationery Office, Dublin.

Shackle, M. (1993) *I Thought I Was the Only One: A Report of a Conference — Disabled People, Pregnancy and Early Parenthood*, Maternity Alliance, London.

Shackle, P. and Ryan, M. (1994) "What is the Role of the Consumer in Health Care?" *Journal of Social Policy*, 23 (4), pp. 517–541.

Sharing in Progress: National Anti-Poverty Strategy (1997), Stationery Office, Dublin.

Shea, D. (1991) *Reproductive Care: Experiences of Some Women Drug Users*. M.A. thesis (Women's Studies), Part fulfilment of M.Phil Degree in Women's Studies.

Sherr, L. (1995) *The Psychology of Pregnancy and Childbirth*, Blackwell Science, Oxford.

Siim, B. (1988) "Towards a Feminist Rethinking of the Welfare State" in Jones, K. and Jonasdottir, A. (eds.) *The Political Interests of Women Developing Theory and Research with a Feminist Face*, Sage, London.

Silverton, L. (1993) *The Art and Science of Midwifery*, Prentice Hall, London.

Simkin, P. (1989) "Non-pharmacological Methods of Pain Relief during Labor", in Chalmers, I. et al. (eds.), *Effective Care in Pregnancy and Childbirth*, Oxford University Press, Oxford.

Simkin, P. and Enkin, M. (1989) "Antenatal Classes" in Chalmers, I. et al. (eds.), *Effective Care in Pregnancy and Childbirth*, Oxford University Press, Oxford.

Siney, C. (1995) (ed.) *The Pregnant Drug Addict*, Books for Midwives Press, England.

Siney, C (1997) *Pregnancy and Drug Misuse* in Kargar, I. and Hunt, S.C. (eds.), *Challenges in Midwifery Care*, Macmillan Press, London, pp. 133–145.

Siney, C. (1999) (ed.) *Pregnancy and Drug Misuse*, Books for Midwives Press. England.

Sloan, D., and O'Connor, J.J. (1998) "The Treatment of Opiate Addiction during Pregnancy", *Irish Medical Journal*, Oct/Nov 1998, Vol. 91, No. 5.

Smaje, C. (1995) *Health, Race and Ethnicity: Making Sense of the Evidence*, King's Fund Institute, London.

Smith, S. (1998) "Women and HIV" in *Women and Health*, Barry, M., Conroy, J., Hayes, A., O'Kelly, A. and Shaughnessy, L. (eds.), *Women's Studies Review, Volume Five*, Women's Studies Centre, National University of Ireland, Galway, pp. 81–90.

Smyth, A. (ed.) (1992) *The Abortion Papers*, Attic, Dublin.

Smyth, A. (ed.) (1993) *Irish Women's Studies Reader*, Attic, Dublin.

Smyth, E. (1997) "Labour Market Structures and Women's Employment in the Republic of Ireland", Byrne, A. and Leonard, M. (eds.),, *Women and Irish Society: A Sociological Reader*, Beyond the Pale, Belfast, pp. 63–80.

Solomons, M. (1969) *Life Cycle: Facts for Adults*, Allen Figgis, Dublin.

Solomons, M. (1992) *Pro Life?* Lilliput Press, Dublin.

Stacey, M. (1988) *The Sociology of Health and Healing*, Routledge, London.

Stanley, L. and Wise, S. (1993) *Breaking Out Again: Feminist Ontology and Epistomology*, Routledge, London.

Stanworth, M. (1987) "The Deconstruction of Motherhood" in Stanworth, M. (ed.), *Reproductive Technologies*, Polity Press, Cambridge.

Stanworth, M. (1994) "Reproductive Technologies", *The Polity Reader in Gender Studies*, Polity Press, Cambridge.

Stocking, B. (1992) "Research Findings and Policy-making" in Chamberlain, G. and Zander, L. (eds.) *Pregnancy Care in the 1990s*, Cromwell Press, Wiltshire.

Stuart, J.J. (1958) *Clinical Report, Coombe Lying-In Hospital*, Dublin.

Suleiman, S.R. (ed.) (1986) *The Female Body in Western Culture: Contemporary Perspectives*, Harvard University Press, London.

Sunstein, C. (ed.) (1990) *Feminism and Political Theory*, University of Chicago Press, London, Chicago.

Swain, J., Finkelstein, V., French, S. and Oliver, M. (eds.) *Disabling Barriers, Enabling Environments*, London, Open University Press/Sage.

Symonds, A. and Hunt, S.C. (1996) *The Midwife and Society: Perspectives, Policies and Practice*, Macmillan, London.

Task Force on the Travelling Community Report (1995), Stationery Office, Dublin.

Taylor-Gooby, P. (1991) "Welfare State Regimes and Welfare Citizenship", *Journal of Social Policy*, 1 (20), pp. 93–105.

Tew, M. (1995) *Safer Childbirth: A Critical History of Maternity Care* (2nd edition), Chapman and Hall, London.

Thomson, A.M. (1989) "Why Don't Women Breastfeed?", in Robinson, S. and Thomson, A.M. (eds.), *Midwives, Research and Childbirth*, Vol. 1, Chapman and Hall, London.

Tierney, M. (1978) *Modern Ireland Revised*, Gill and Macmillan, Dublin.

Towards an Independent Future: Report of the Review Group on Health and Social Services for People with Physical and Sensory Disabilities (1996), Stationery Office, Dublin.

UNICEF, *The State of the World's Children*, Oxford University Press, Oxford.

Valiulis, M.G. (1997) "Engendering Citizenship: Women's Relationship to the State in Ireland and the United States in the Post-Suffrage Period", in Valiulis, M.G. and O'Dowd, M. (eds.), *Women and Irish History*, Wolfhound Press, Dublin, pp. 159–172.

Van Buren, J.S. (1989) *The Modernist Madonna: Semiotics of the Maternal Metaphor*, Karnac, London.

Van der Kam, S. (2000) "Mental Health Needed for Caring Capacity" *Field Exchange*, Issue 9, March, pp. 8–9.

Van Esterik, P. (1989) *Motherpower and Infant Feeding*, Zed Books, London.

Van Every, J. (1991) "Who is the Family? The Assumptions of British Social Policy", *Critical Social Policy*, Issue 33, Winter 1991/1992, pp. 62–75.

Waddell, S. (1992) *High Chairs and Children*, Words Work, New Zealand.

Wagner, M. (1994) *Pursuing the Birth Machine: The Search for Appropriate Birth Technology*, ACE Graphics, Sevenoaks, Kent.

Wagner, M. (1995) *Appropriate Birth Technology: Getting It Right*, Paper delivered at Reclaiming Birth Seminar, Queens University Belfast, June.

Walby, S. (1990) *Theorizing Patriarchy*, Basil Blackwell, Oxford.

Walsh Noonan, P. (2002) "Women's Health: A Conceptual Approach" in Walsh Noonan, P. and Heller, T., *Health of Women with Intellectual Disabilities*, Blackwell, Oxford, pp. 7–21.

Walsh Noonan, P. and Heller, T. (2002) *Health of Women with Intellectual Disabilities*, Blackwell, Oxford.

Ward, M. (1983) *Unmanageable Revolutionaries: Women and Irish Nationalism*, Brandon, Dingle, Co. Kerry.

Wates, M. (1997) *Disabled Parents: Dispelling the Myths*, a National Childbirth Trust Guide, UK.

Weeks, J. and Holland, J. (1996) *Sexual Cultures, Communities, Values and Intimacy*, Macmillan, Basingstoke.

Wegar, K. (1997) "In Search of Bad Mothers: Social Constructions of Birth and Adoptive Motherhood", *Women's Studies International Forum*, Pergamon, Vol. 20, No. 1, pp. 77–86.

Weingrad Smith, J. and Tully, M.R. (2001) "Midwifery Management of Breastfeeding: Using the Evidence", *Journal of Midwifery and Women's Health*, Vol. 46, No. 6, November/December, pp. 423–438.

Wells, P.N.T. (1987a) "The Safety of Diagnostic Ultrasound: Report of a British Institute of Radiology Working Group", *British Journal of Radiology*, Supplement No. 20.

Wells, P.N.T. (1987b) "The Prudent Use of Diagnostic Ultrasound", *Ultrasound in Medicine and Biology*, 13 (7), pp. 391–400.

Wesson, N. (1995a) *Alternative Maternity* (revised edition), Optima, London.

Wesson, N. (1995b) *Home Birth: A Practical Guide*, Optima, London.

WHO (1985a) *Having a Baby in Europe*, Public Health in Europe, 26, WHO Regional Office for Europe, Copenhagen.

WHO (1985b) *WHO Consensus Conference on Appropriate Technology for Birth, Fortaleza, Brazil, 22–26 April, 1985, Summary Report*, WHO Regional Office for Europe, Copenhagen.

WHO (1988) *The Partograph: A Managerial Tool for the Prevention of Prolonged Labour*, WHO/MCH/88.3, Geneva.

WHO (1991a) *Maternal Mortality Rates and Ratios* (3rd edition), Safe Motherhood Programme, WHO, Geneva.

WHO (1991b) *Postnatal Depression: A Review*, European Regional Office, Copenhagen.

WHO (2001) *New Data on the Prevention of Mother-to-Child Transmission of HIV and Their Policy Implications: Conclusions and Recommendations*, WHO Technical Consultation on Behalf of the UNFPA/UNICEF/WHO/UN AIDS Inter-Agency Task Team on Mother to Child Transmission of HIV, Geneva.

WHO/UNICEF (1990) *Protecting, Promoting and Supporting Breastfeeding: The Special Role of Maternity Services*, Geneva.

Whyte, J. (1980) *Church and State in Modern Ireland, 1923–1979*, Gill and Macmillan, Dublin.

Wilding, P. (1994) "Maintaining Quality in Human Services", *Social Policy and Administration*, Vol. 28, No. 1, March.

Wiley, M. and Merriman, B. (1996) *Women and Health Care in Ireland: Knowledge, Attitudes and Behaviour*, Oak Tree Press in association with ESRI, Dublin.

Williams, F. (1989) *Social Policy: A Critical Introduction, Issues of Race, Gender and Class*, Polity, Cambridge.

Williams, M. and Booth, D. (1984) *Antenatal Education: Guidelines for Teachers* (2nd edition), Churchill Livingstone, Edinburgh.

Wilson, E. (1977) *Women and the Welfare State*, Tavistock, London.

Windebank, J. (1996) "To What Extent Can Social Policy Challenge the Dominant Ideology of Mothering? A Cross-national Comparison of Sweden, France and Britain", *Journal of European Social Policy*, 6 (2), pp. 147–161.

Wistow, G. and Henwood, M. (1990–1991) "Caring for People: Elegant Model or Flawed Design", *Social Policy Review 1990–1991*, Social Policy Association, pp. 78–100.

Women's Health Unit (2001) *The National Maternity Hospital Domino and Hospital Outreach Home Birth Service Pilot Project Evaluation*, Dublin: Women's Health Unit, Northern Area Health Board.

Woods, M. and Humphries, N. (2001) *Statistical Update: Seeking Asylum in Ireland*, Applied Social Science Research Programme, UCD Dublin.

Zweifler, J. and Gonzalez, A.M. (1998) "Teaching Residents to Care for Culturally Diverse Populations", *Academic Medicine*, Vol. 73, No. 10, October, pp. 1056–1061.

INDEX